New Procedures in Spinal Interventional Neuroradiology

Series Editor
Luigi Manfrè

For further volumes: http://www.springer.com/series/13394

Luigi Manfrè
Editor

Spinal Canal Stenosis

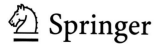 Springer

Editor
Luigi Manfrè
Minimal Invasive Spine Therapy
Cannizzaro Hospital
Catania, Italy

Electronic supplementary material is available in the online version of chapter 2 on SpringerLink: http://link.springer.com

ISBN 978-3-319-26268-0   ISBN 978-3-319-26270-3   (eBook)
DOI 10.1007/978-3-319-26270-3

Library of Congress Control Number: 2016938231

Printed on acid-free paper

This Springer imprint is published by Springer Nature
The registered company is Springer International Publishing AG Switzerland

Contents

Imaging and Symptoms of Spinal Canal Stenosis

Cosma Andreula, Gianpiero Berardi,
and Alessandra Tripoli

Spinal canal stenosis is a *unisegmental* or *polysegmental* narrowing of the central spinal canal and/or of the lateral recesses and/or of the root canals which can lead to nerve roots or spinal cord compression. This condition is more common in the cervical and lumbar tracts.

Patients with cervical spinal stenosis have insidious onset symptoms, characterized by uni- or bilateral radiculopathy or myelopathy, (e.g., gait disturbance progressive paraparesis related, dysesthesias). Cervical pain is often associated with spinal canal strictness and constriction, but it is not specific. In particular, cervical stenosis may be limited to a simple radiculopathy, with radicular pain, which radiates along the corresponding dermatome, combined with acute painful crisis and functional limitation of neck flexion (Fig. 1.1).

Sometimes, though, the stenosis can bring to a slow and progressive compression in the spinal cord, in the small medullary vessels, and also in the anterior spinal artery (which supplies blood to the anterior two-third of the spinal cord).

Thus was the true myelopathy which is characterized by a clinical picture that, in most cases, can be described as follows: after a long period of painful radicular paresthesias in neck (with functional limitation of the neck), shoulder, and upper limb, caused by neck movements (radicular pains phase), autonomic disorders appear due to cervical sympathetic pain (hyperhidrosis, hypothermia, edema) and disorders of movement both sympathetic and peripheral.

Generally, the former are in the lower limbs and can even bring to spastic paraplegia (impairment of the pyramidal system); the latter, the peripheral ones,

C. Andreula, M.D. (✉) • A. Tripoli
Unit of Radiology and Neuroradiology, Anthea Hospital, Bari, Italy
e-mail: cosma.andreula@gmail.com

G. Berardi
Unit of Radiology, The Accredited Private Hospital S. Maria, Bari, Italy

© Springer International Publishing Switzerland 2016
L. Manfrè (ed.), *Spinal Canal Stenosis*, New Procedures in Spinal Interventional
Neuroradiology, DOI 10.1007/978-3-319-26270-3_1

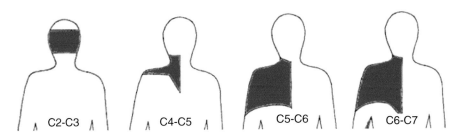

Fig. 1.1 Cervical dermatomes

consisting of hypomuscular atrophies and absence of proprioceptive reflexes, are located in the upper limbs.

There are also lateralized thermodolorific hypoanesthesia (compression on the backs of a spinothalamic bundle) and sphincter disturbances [1–4].

Sometimes, the myelopathic picture is that of a half section of the spinal cord, like Brown-Sequard syndrome, with spastic paralysis (lesion of the pyramidal tracts) and abolition of deep sensitivity, tactile epicritical (lesion of the posterior column), ipsilateral to the lesion, thermal anesthesia, and pain contralateral to the lesion and total anesthesia (radicular lesions or posterior horns) ipsilateral to the lesion, with hyperesthesia over the lesion (lesion of spinothalamic tracts).

But it is also possible to observe clinical patterns of *medullary transverse section* characterized by complete flaccid paraplegia/quadriplegia, pronounced muscular hypotonia, cutaneous and tendon reflexes absence, global sublesional anesthesia, fecal and urinary retention, impossibility of erection and ejaculation, trophic changes of the skin and muscles, absence of sweating, and vasomotor paralysis with arterial hypotension and hypothermia. An accurate early diagnosis is essential, since there is no spontaneous regression of the process and the surgery prevents the progression of symptoms. The stenosis *below* the level of the *conus medullaris* can manifest in many symptoms due to the compression of a single root or the cauda equine and causes pain (at the site of the stenosis and/or irradiated in the limbs), with possible sensory and/or motor deficits. Obviously, the clinical pattern will depend on the extent and on the level of stenosis itself. Since the spinal cord usually ends at the level of the lower border of the vertebra L1, the lumbosacral roots, to reach the foramen where they exit from the spinal canal, must move downward obliquely, touching anteriorly with the intervertebral disks, with the interposition of the posterior longitudinal ligament. So it is clear that if the stenosis involves only the intervertebral foramen, it will compress the roots with the name of the lower vertebra, but if it also leads to a reduction of the anteroposterior diameter, it can also compress one or more underlying roots [1–4] (Fig. 1.2).

So the pain can be either root or spinal. Radicular pain is generally of sciatica type since it is linked to the compression of the roots that give rise to the sciatic nerve (L5, S1, S2, etc.), but can also be a cruralgia type in cases where also L4 root, a root that gives rise to the femoral nerve, is compressed.

Fig. 1.2 In the lumbar tract radicular compression can involve the foramen or the underlying roots of the cauda

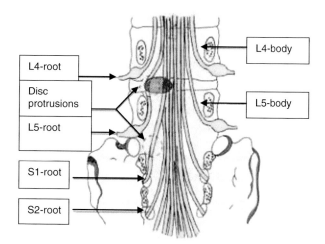

Radicular pain is localized in the site of innervation of the compressed root; generally it is not continuous and can be exacerbated by situations that accentuate the compression or stretching of the same root; typically, upright position with the straight leg, coughing, sneezing, and straining are all situations that result in an increase in CSF pressure resulting in higher compression on the nerve roots.

The Lasègue sign, in patients with lumbar canal stenosis, is positive in both phases; particularly pain is evoked with the patient supine, both during flexion of the thigh on the pelvis to leg extended, both during flexion of the thigh on the pelvis bent leg. The extent of root compression determines the extent of pain within the dermatome and then the different degree of positivity of the Lasègue sign. The intensity of the pain varies according to the degree of extension of the leg on the thigh.

The pains of the spine are localized, instead, in the lumbosacral region (low back pain); they don't have a provision root, are exacerbated by finger pressure exerted in the paravertebral site (signs of Delitala, Lasègue, and Valleix), in correspondence of the intervertebral disk, and are often associated with stiffness of the lumbar spine, with obvious limitation of any movement of the trunk [1–4]. The lumbar spine is stiff, the back muscles are contracted. In the upright position, the pelvis is tilting towards the healthy side with compensatory and analgesic scoliosis. From a pathophysiological point of view, low back pain is the clinical expression of the stretch of the peripheral portion of the fibrous ring that along with other structures (such as the posterior longitudinal ligament, capsular ligament structures of the vertebral joints, etc.) is innervated by branches of breast – spinal nerve Luschka.

The typical symptoms of stenosis are therefore a direct result of the compression of the spinal roots and can affect one or both legs. The main symptom is pain in the legs that is frequently associated to low back pain.

The pain in the lower limbs is generally slight at rest but becomes increasingly evident with ambulation, until the patient is forced to stop. The stop determines the attenuation of pain but reappears after another route; in advanced stages, the duration of ambulation is reduced more and more, forcing the patient to more frequent stops ("disease of the showcases"). This typical phenomenon is called intermittent neurogenic "claudication" and is distinguished from the similar symptoms of vascular origin (arterial vascular disease of the lower limbs), as it is not associated with pale skin, hypothermia, and decrease in periferal arterial pulses.

The *symptoms are intermittent and therefore manifest only* when the nerve roots are compressed, with the erect posture and gait; this means that often, in the root canal stenosis, moderate, electromyographic findings are normal or uncharacteristic.

Disordered sensitivity is located in the site of innervation of the root and suffering can be irritative (paresthesias) or deficient (numbness). The motor disorders can range from mild weakness to a paresis important with atrophy of muscles innervated by the root tablet. A sign that may be present in addition, regardless of the presence of motor deficits, is the reduction of tendon reflexes.

Sometimes, the clinical pattern is dominated by motor deficits when the anterior motor roots are mainly compressed.

When many roots are compressed, bilaterally cauda equina syndrome (compression of the spinal nerve roots that emerge below the first lumbar root) can emerge, with lower back pain and pain radiated to the thighs, the legs, the perineum, with hypesthesia or saddle anesthesia also extended to the posteroexternal part of the legs and back of the foot and motor deficits (which may vary, depending on the roots compressed, by a deficiency of the flexion and extension of the foot and toes to a flaccid paralysis with atrophy of the leg muscles also, foot of the buttock and thigh posteriorly). Sphincter deficiency and sexual impotency may also be present [1–5].

In etiopathogenetic terms, stenosis is distinguished in:

- Congenital stenosis (idiopathic, spondyloepiphyseal dysplasia from strength from vitamin D, achondroplasia, mucopolysaccharidosis): they present with short and stubby peduncles, shortness of the sagittal and interpedicular diameter, hypertrophy, and verticalization of the laminae; the spinal canal appears small, as well as reduced, until with the complete absence, appears the epidural fat. The achondroplasia is a congenital autosomal dominant disease (gene mapped to the short arm of chromosome 4, 16.3 locus, which encodes the receptor for fibroblast growth factor (FGF)), which leads to poor response to the stimulus of osteogenic growth plates. It is a disease characterized by rhizomelic dwarfism (small growth in length of the upper and lower limbs, particularly with respect to the proximal bone, in the absence of deficit of the trunk); kyphosis at the thoracolumbar transition, reducing the distance interpedicular descending toward skull (caudal); vertebral bodies with flattened stalks abnormal short hand ("trident") with II, III, and IV finger courts and of the same length; and alteration of the hinge craniomegaly C0–C2. With time, the congenital stenosis may overlap degenerative joint interpeduncular and structures intervertebral disc structures, which aggravates the clinical condition [5–11].

Mucopolysaccharidosis is a congenital disease related to several enzyme deficiencies involved in the catabolism of mucopolysaccharides, resulting in accumulation of these macromolecules in various parts of the body. Affected individuals are stocky characterized by facial features, and also with hepatosplenomegaly, umbilical hernia, and multiplex dysostosis skeletal dysostosis. At the spinal level, odontoid hypoplasia occurs with thickening of the transverse ligament of the tooth in relation to the deposition of mucopolysaccharides, multiple disk protrusion, biconvex deformation, and oval or rectangular shape of the vertebral bodies, which have beaks protruding at the corners of vertebral bodies. Dural thickening and yellow ligaments can present too [6].

Acquired stenosis: they can be a result of surgery, injury, trauma, neoplasm, but above all, degenerative changes of the vertebral bodies (spondylosis, osteophytes), of the articular masses (osteochondrosis, osteoarthritis), intervertebral disk (protrusion, rear disk herniation), of the yellow ligaments (hyperplasia, calcification by degeneration), and/or of the posterior longitudinal ligament (ossification). The same reduction in the height of the intervertebral space, from disk degeneration, can cause the shortening and thickening of the intervertebral ligaments, and consequent imprint on the dural sac. In most cases, the acquired stenosis evolves from a condition of disk degeneration resulting in protrusion of the annulus fibrosus, which is accompanied by phenomena of osteophytes and spondylosis of vertebral bodies corresponding to the load, with an initial narrowing of the canal root canal [5–11].

The biomechanical overload resulting from these changes affects the interapophyseal joints, which develop degenerative arthritic phenomena, characterized by osteophytic protrusions hypertrophy and osteosclerotical thickening of the subchondral facet joints, which, in periods of exacerbation, may present hydrarthrosis. In this phase of etiopathogenesis, an extension of the root canal narrowing to both posterolateral recesses usually occurs. The altered mechanical stress and the local phlogogenic stimulation extend finally to yellow ligament (overexpressing certain receptors for growth factors such as TGFβ), determining hypertrophy, with narrowing of the spinal canal and posterior symmetrical full-blown picture of stenosis (Fig. 1.3). The process can get to spondylolisthesis caused by instability of the interapophyseal joints [5–11].

Mixed stenosis: they are the most frequent in clinical practice and are derived from the overlap of an acquired form of congenital stenosis; in this case, a disk or osteophyte protrusion, even slight, can lead to severe or radicular compression of the dural sac.

Under the topographic profile, stenoses are divided into:

- Central: they are characterized by a reduction in size of the central spinal canal that in degenerative forms is supported by the disk protrusion, from hyperplasia and/or calcification of the yellow ligaments and the hypertrophy and degenerative joint osteophytes of the masses.
- Lateral: they include stenosis of the lateral recesses and of the root canals.

Stenosis of the lateral recesses that result in changes ("cloverleaf") (trefoil) of the spinal canal is due to hypertrophy with degenerative joint osteophytes of the masses. Sometimes, this may be unilateral, although in most cases, it is bilateral and symmetrical. Due to a stricture agenesis that can be represented by a synovial cyst from an interapophyseal joint [5–11].

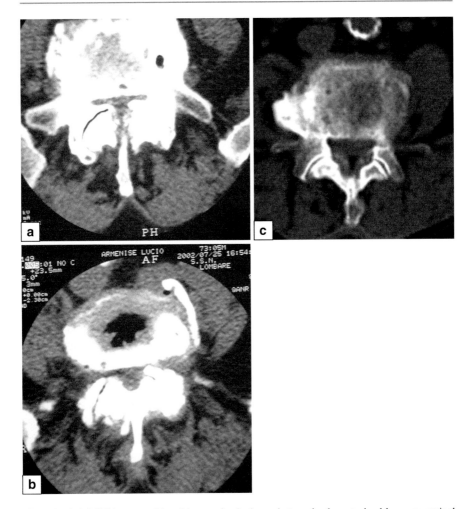

Fig. 1.3 Axial CT images with evidence of spinal canal stenosis characterized by symmetrical arthritis and osteophytosis of intervertebral joints (**a, b**), with gas-vacuolar degeneration (**a**), hypertrophy of the yellow ligament, with associated contextual calcified spots (**a, c**)

Stenosis of root canals, more frequent than the last one, is mostly supported by congenital factors (shortness of peduncle): by disk protrusion and posterolateral osteophytes of vertebral bodies.

1.1 Physiopathology

The degenerative phenomena of diskoligamentous and bony elements are the most common causes of spinal stenosis that, in the lumbar tract, most frequently involve the levels L4–L5 and L5–S1.

The spine, as already said, is to be considered as a dynamic complex constituted by a single functional unit, whose components are interrelated and interdependent.

Having said that, it is clear that the physiological and progressive degenerative dehydration of intervertebral disk determines an overstrain of facet joints and, consequently, suffering degenerative factors latter determines an overstrain of disk – somatic joint.

The various static and dynamic stresses, especially stress rotary, involve disk degeneration and facet joint. It follows protrusion and reduction in height of the disk, limiting approach and sclerosis of the vertebral osteophyte formations with stenosis of the central channel, subluxation in upward and forward of the superior articular masses resulting in stenosis of the lateral recesses and of the root canals [5–7, 9–11].

The alterations of the articular masses include sclerosis and hypertrophy, loss of articular cartilage, subchondral vacuoles, osteophytes, and subluxation resulting in degenerative spondylolisthesis.

Degenerative spondylolisthesis, more frequent in the L4–L5, involves a compression of the dural sac between the posterior arch of the vertebra above given that slides forward and the vertebral body below (bayonet mechanism).

Even degenerative changes of no bony structures can be due to spinal stenosis. An annulus fibrosus protrusion reduces the sagittal diameter of the spinal canal central, but it can also lead to stenosis of the lateral recesses or root canal and thickening of the ligaments yellow, due to fibrosis in fatty infiltration or calcific deposits, reduces the transverse diameter of the rear portion of the center channel and also reduces the sagittal diameter displacing forward the dural sac.

1.2   Radiographic Examination

The radiographic examination, if of good technical quality, shows the degenerative changes, but it is not able to make an accurate diagnosis [11–19]. A spinal canal of normal size may be stenotic for the thickening of the ligamentous components. Furthermore, measurements of the diameters of the spinal canal are not very reliable, given the considerable individual variability, especially in the lumbar tract. It is true, however, that at the cervical level, there are two reference semiological radiographs to assess the magnitude of the sagittal diameter of the spinal canal: the first corresponds to the line that runs along the posterior margin of the vertebral bodies; the second is constituted by the spinolaminar line. This imaginary line combines together the points of convergence of the laminae of each vertebral body in the midline, at the plant of the spinous processes. Normally, the spinolaminar line is convex in the anterior part and separates, at least 3–4 mm, from the posterior edge of the articular masses. If the spinolaminar line is to overlap the mass joints, you can, with absolute certainty, infer that the sagittal diameter of the cervical spinal canal is reduced, provided of course there is articular malposition of the masses [1–4] (Fig. 1.4).

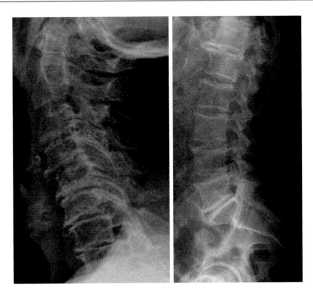

Fig. 1.4 Prescription in patients with cervical spondylosis lumbar advanced degree. Spinal stenosis is conceivable but poorly demonstrable

A lumbar conventional radiography of the spine can detect phenomena of spondylosis and interapophyseal osteoarthritis which are crucial determinants in the onset of root canal stenosis. The interapophyseal joints, in particular, can be measured both in the lateral projection and in the frontal one, appearing thickened and hypertrophic. The lateral projection also allows to highlight osteophytic protrusions along the edges of somatic posterior vertebral limiting. However, standard radiographs do not allow a direct assessment of the anatomical structures that make up the walls and osteoarticular ligaments of the vertebral canal [1–4, 11, 19].

Conventional radiography, with the lateral projection, can highlight the so-called spondylolisthesis, that is, an alteration of the metateric alignment characterized by ventral slippage of a vertebra compared to the one below, indicating an advanced arthritic process, with instability of the interapophyseal facet joints as a late complication. This condition must be distinguished from isthmic spondylolysis, that is, a ventral slippage of vertebral body compared to the vertebra below, caused by the bilateral interruption of the vertebral arch at the isthmus. The two processes can be discriminated against, in the lateral projection, using the so-called sign of the spinous process (of Bryk and Rosenkranz).

In summary, in listhesis caused by isthmic lysis, the vertebral body will slide forward and not the corresponding spinous process; it follows that in a lateral projection, its lack of alignment with the other spinous processes above will determine the formation of a step located above the level of spondylolisthesis. On the contrary, in the case of degenerative spondylolisthesis, the entire vertebra (including the spinous process) will slide forward and, in a lateral projection, the step of nonalignment of the spinous processes will be formed below the level of listhesis [11, 19, 20].

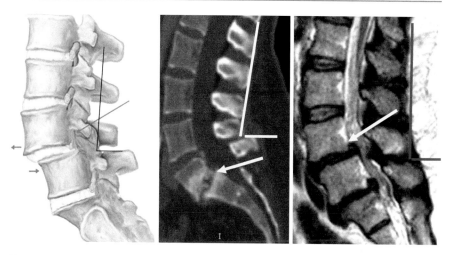

Fig. 1.5   A sign of the spinous process (of Bryk and Rosenkranz). The figure on the *left* and the T2-weighted image sagittal MRI *right*, the misalignment of the spinous processes is located below the spondylolisthesis, degenerative basis. In the central image TC, misalignment occurs to it above the spondylolisthesis, which in this case depends on the isthmic lysis

However, these semiological subtleties collide in clinical practice, with poor reliability of the metameric alignment, especially in patients with lumbar scoliosis sometimes secondary to degenerative processes and advanced with the technical difficulties in the proper delineation of the spinous processes in the lateral view. Isthmic lysis can be classically detected by oblique projections with the "Scottish doggie sign," but even then, with the advent of multislice CT with multiplanar reconstructions, this finding presents a relative significance in the differential diagnosis between isthmic lysis and spondylolisthesis instability (Fig. 1.5).

1.3   TC

CT is essential in the precise evaluation of the causes of degenerative spinal stenosis, since it well documents the somatic and facet joints of osteoproductive processes, the degenerative changes of intervertebral disks, hyperplasia of yellow ligament (only in the lumbar spine), and/or their calcification [6, 8–13] .

The TC, therefore, evaluates very well the state of the whole osteo-disk-ligament case (Fig. 1.6).

In case of degenerative spondylolisthesis, CT identifies easily subluxation of the interapophyseal facet joints, the sign of "double arch," and in the sagittal multiplanar reconstructions, "bayonet" deformation of the dural sac.

The method also allows, better than MRI, an easy measurement of the diameters of the spinal canal. Median sagittal diameters <10 mm are indicative of absolute root canal stenosis, while values between 10 and 13 mm indicate a condition of incipient narrowing.

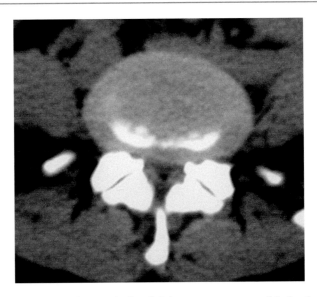

Fig. 1.6 TC identifies posterior vertebral arch joint structures responsible for the stenosis and allows you to determine their amount. In addition, the method allows a good view of the yellow ligaments and intervertebral disk. However, the display of the contents of the spinal canal is limited compared to the RM

However, the measurement of the sagittal diameter in the median region is not as reliable, especially if the degenerative phenomena involve predominantly the inter-apophyseal joints with prevailing narrowing of the lateral recesses. Also, it is to be considered pathognomonic of the central spinal stenosis, not so much the reduction in size of the channel expressed in millimeters, as the disappearance of the epidural fat. Considering also the congenital conditions of shortening of the pedicles, absolute measurements of the diameters root canal can be misleading for the correct definition of stenosis [6, 8–13].

In this regard, various criteria for measuring diameters of root canal have been proposed by several authors. The Jones-Thompson quotient, for example, quantifies the root canal stenosis respectively dividing the product of interpedicular distance (A) to the maximum anteroposterior diameter of the spinal canal (B), with the product of the maximum transverse diameter (C) and anteroposterior maximum (D) of the disk. $A \times B / C \times D$ has a v. n. > 4.5. Values below this threshold are considered pathological. In this case, however, the RM is better suited to the measurement of the TC of different diameters used for the calculation of the quotient, ensuring a better delineation of the annulus fibrosus disk. Other authors have linked the overall reduction of the surface area of the dural sac (with values < 75 mm ^ 2), and the onset of painful symptoms in patients with narrow channel compared to normal subjects, the values of area surface were never less than 128 mm ^ 2 [11] (Fig. 1.7).

In the daily clinical-radiological experience, measurements of this kind, as quality, are of limited use for their complexity, and what is more important for the correct detection of stenosis is the assessment of containing (vertebral canal) and the

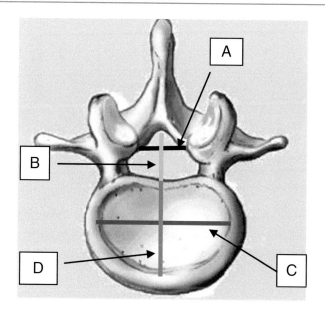

Fig. 1.7 Calculation of the quotient of Jones-Thompson. The black line indicates the interpedicular distance (A). The *green line* indicates the maximum anteroposterior diameter of the channel (B). The *red line* (C) indicates the maximum transverse diameter of the disk interspace. The blue line (D) indicates the maximum anteroposterior diameter of the disk interspace

content (lots of dural and spinal nerve roots) in different spaces of interbody evaluated comparatively, level by level, according to the axial planes.

CT, however, is not able to identify the effects of the disease on the spinal extradural determines. Moreover, in the cervical spine, the low amount of epidural fat and its small size of the spinal canal are insufficient to assess a possible ligamentous hypertrophy [5, 6, 11–13] (Fig. 1.8).

1.4 RM

There is no doubt that the RM presents undeniable advantages over CT in the analysis of the relationship between "contains" and "content" spine. It demonstrates optimal phenomena of compression on the spinal cord (myelo RM), their extension (panning direct sagittal), and, above all, the effect on the nervous structures and the possible suffering of the latter (edema, gliosis, and myelomalacia marrow). These advantages mean that, especially in the cervical spine, MRI represents the preferred method of screening [6, 13, 15] (Fig. 1.9).

The radicular compression is indicated, in the sagittal T1 dependent, by the dislocation or disappearance of periradicular fat; compression of the dural sac and disk degeneration, however, are more evident in the images of T2 – dependent. The T2*-dependent images identify osteophytes and differentiate them from an adjacent herniating disk tissue [21]. Furthermore, especially in the cervical spine, they clearly

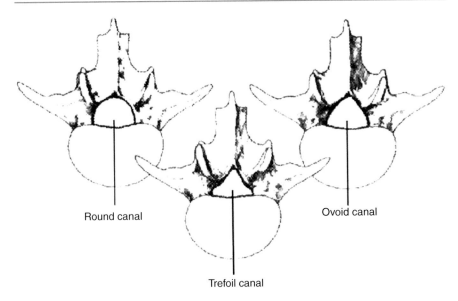

Round canal   Trefoil canal   Ovoid canal

Fig. 1.8 Different morphologies of the spinal canal in relation to anatomic variations of the vertebral bodies: round, clover, ovoid

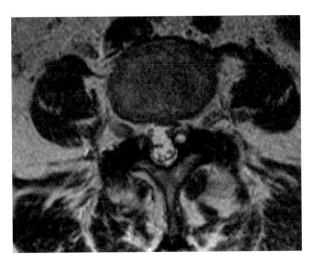

Fig. 1.9 Rare case of bilateral interapophyseal, synovial cyst, determining root canal stenosis and well detectable with MRI sequences axial T2 weighted

demonstrate the ossification of the posterior longitudinal ligament and yellow ligament hypertrophy because of the high contrast that exists between these structures and the adjacent subarachnoid space.

In the images, axial T1 and T2 MRI identifies employees "clover" morphology of the spinal canal, which, unlike the other anatomical round and oval variants, predisposes to the onset of the stenosis [5, 6, 13–15].

The yellow ligaments can be well defined and their hypertrophy (7–8 mm thick compared to normal values that do not exceed 4 mm) is reflected in a typical bilateral and symmetric protrusion of the ligamentous borders, with narrowing of the posterior vertebral canal. Always through the axial images, T1- and T2-weighted MRI allow an accurate study of the lateral recesses, of phenomena of degenerative joint disease, and interapophyseal chondropathy associated with them; the latter is much more visible than the TC due to intrinsic most contrast resolution of the method.

In this regard, a possible cause of the acute symptoms is represented by the formation of synovial cysts that protrude into the spinal canal and lateral recesses, compressing the nerve roots. These injuries can be easily attributed to "space-occupying" synovial protrusions, thanks to RM, which, through its multiplanar capabilities and its excellent contrast resolution, defines the signal and the morphology and distinguishes the contours of the nerve root through sagittal T2-weighted images [5, 6, 13–15, 22, 23]. These acquisition plans also allow to appreciate the obliteration of the epidural fat that surrounds the nerve root, which is also a sign of lateral compression (Fig. 1.10).

MRI also allows to identify phenomena of nerve root compression by the vertebral pedicles, related to thinning asymmetric disk interspace. This framework, which the Anglo-Saxon authors label as "pedicular kinking," takes place in the event of severe disk degeneration – somatic asymmetric, when the vertebra above the slender portion laterally to the left or right of a disk interspace tilts caudally, approaching the vertebra below. This involves a descent of the corresponding stalk that contacts the nerve root. This phenomenon, commonly found in the lumbar spine, especially in elderly patients who have scoliotic deviations secondary to spondylosis and arthrosis interapophyseal, is properly documented with T1- and T2-weighted coronal plane, with which you can have direct visualization of the sacral plexus [5].

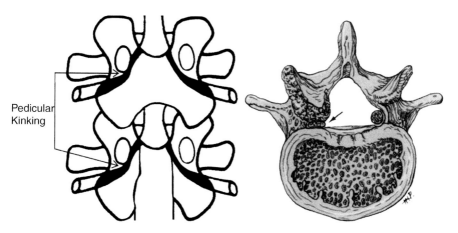

Pedicular
Kinking

Fig. 1.10 Possible causes of stenosis asymmetric with nerve root compression: the image on the *right* shows the phenomenon of pedicular kinking, the *left* hip osteoarthritis

MRI also enables an optimal and essential evaluation of the spinal "content." In the neck, in fact, the myelomalacia, with focal areas of hyperintensity on T2-weighted medulla, centrally located, with irregular margins and placed in the stricture, is a pathognomonic sign of medullary suffering. In order to differentiate the areas of myelomalacia from the gliosis, the T1-weighted sagittal plane is of considerable importance. The areas of myelomalacia, in fact, are hypointense T1 lesions, while gliotic lesions appear little or no distinguishable in these sequences [6, 13, 15, 21].

In this regard, FLAIR-T1 weighted sequences have recently been developed, which broke down the signal of CSF, allowing better delineation of the spinal cord and epidural space. The best resulting anatomical detail ensures optimal evaluation of containing and content, essential for the correct interpretation of the images and their correlation with the clinical pattern. These sequences also are less affected by any artifacts from magnetic susceptibility compared not only to the sequences to echo gradient but also against the same sequences to spin echo, benefiting from the prepulse reversal of MML to 180 °, which provides an additional recovery phase coherence to spin. As in all the T1-weighted sequences, even in FLAIR T1, there has been a marked improvement in the quality iconographic in terms of S/N ratio with increasing magnetic field, so these sequences are used widely in the devices at high field (3 T) [15, 16, 21, 24].

At the axial plane, the cervical spine is preferable to use T2 to echo gradient, which provide an optimal anatomical detail of the spinal cord, differentiating the gray matter (anterior and posterior horns and commissure) from the white (front, rear, and side cords). These sequences are particularly useful in the context of bone marrow disease, in differentiating the various pathological conditions in relation to the topography of the lesion (e.g., back cords in immune-mediated inflammatory lesions such as multiple sclerosis, compared to front cords involved in myelomalacia derived from canal stenosis) [15, 16, 21, 24] (Fig. 1.11).

Recently, Kang, Lee, and other authors have tested a grading for the evaluation of cervical stenosis, using T2-weighted images in the sagittal plane, based on four levels: (1) absence of central stenosis, (2) obliteration of the subarachnoid space in the absence of deformation of the bone marrow, (3) obliteration of the subarachnoid space with medullary deformation, and (4) myelomalacia. This approach, although suggestive, presents some critical points. Infact con "the study, which is retrospective" conducted does not allow to correlate adequately RM alterations emerged at the time of the survey with the symptomatology reported by patients enrolled and limits the latter not particularly significant in cases of overt myelomalacia, but rather in the less severe degrees of stenosis. Moreover, this model, while describing various degrees of stenosis, does not provide reliable predictors on how much and how long a certain stage can evolve into the next [14] (Fig. 1.12).

The spinal content, in the lumbar seat, is represented by the terminal cone and by the cauda equina. Similar to what happens in the cervical tract, also in the lumbar column, such structures are to be well studied with MRI, which can highlight, in the sagittal T2-weighted sequences, the jumble of roots of the cauda equina, which have a convoluted and serpiginous course, at the point of greatest stenosis or a little more cranially to it (Fig. 1.13).

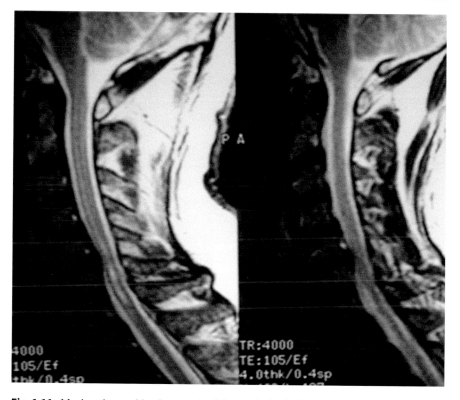

Fig. 1.11 Myelopathy resulting in stenosis of the cervical spinal canal

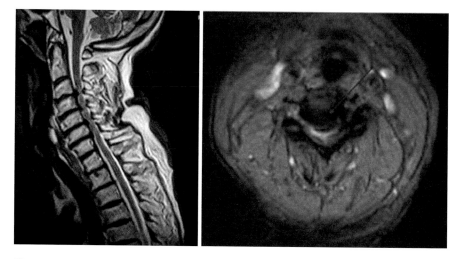

Fig. 1.12 In sagittal T2 will appreciate the extent of stenosis and myelomalacia, in axial T2*, they highlight well the herniated disk, the osteophytes, and hypertrophy of the yellow ligaments *(red arrow)*

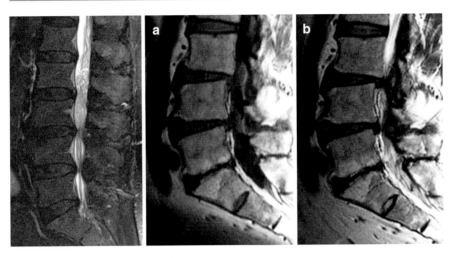

Fig. 1.13 Stenosis of the spinal canal in the lower back causes damage to the roots of the cauda equina, which are well marked with MR acquisitions in the sagittal plane

The use of contrast medium RM is not necessary for the diagnosis of stenosis root canal, as the set of numerous morphostructural alterations of the vertebral canal and of the spinal content is well detectable by the base sequences. However, the contrast agent finds its rationale in all cases in which the root canal stenosis is associated to findings doubts that require differential diagnosis.

It's the case, for example, of the asymmetry of the nerve roots through the intervertebral foramen which have to be differentiated from expansive processes of the same (schwannomas). Furthermore, the expansive neoplastic alterations of the vertebral bodies (somatic metastases, pedicle or more rarely tumors with osteogenic or chondrogenic matrix) must be identified and possibly also characterized with the aid of the contrast medium and with the integration by CT and/or nuclear medicine. Finally, an exacerbation of clinical symptoms related to stenosis can be related to interpedicular inflammation, sometimes asymmetrical, which is well documented by the enhancement of the concerned interapophyseal joint, especially when the existing interapophyseal osteoarthritis is symmetrical and not predominant between the two articular complexes (Fig. 1.14).

The imaging methods described above are not only needed for the diagnostic definition and for the grading of degenerative spinal canal stenosis, but play a crucial role in the choice of a rational possible surgical option. In this regard, it should be noted that this therapeutic approach is not always conclusive and must take into account the preliminary and essential information that both the TC with regard to skeletal component and the phenomena of soft tissue calcification and that the RM with regard to the evaluation of component disks, capsular ligament, and joint and on the content of the spinal canal allow to obtain.

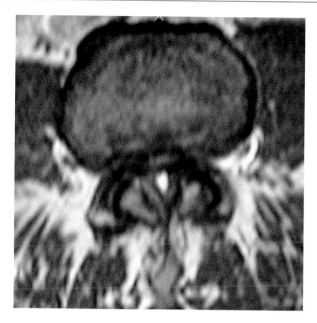

Fig. 1.14 MRI in T1, the axial, highlights the obliteration of the epidural adipose plan resulting herniated disk, as well as detect the hypertrophy of the yellow ligaments and intervertebral joints

References

1. Dorwart RH, Vogler JB, Helms CA. Computed tomography of spinal stenosis. Radiol Clin North Am. 1983;21:301.
2. Kirkaldy-Willis WH, Wedge JH, Yong-Hing K, et al. Pathology and pathogenesis of lumbar spondylosis and stenosis. Spine. 1978;3:319.
3. Modic MT, Masaryk T, Boumphrey F, et al. Lumbar herniated disk disease and canal stenosis: prospective evaluation by surface coil MR, CT, and myelography. AJR. 1986;147:757.
4. Modic MT, Steinberg PM, Ross JS, et al. Degenerative disk disease: assessment of change in vertebral body marrow with MR imaging. Radiology. 1988;166:193.
5. Botwin KP, Gruber RD. Lumbar spinal stenosis, anatomy and pathogenesis. Phys Med Rehabil Clin N Am. 2003;14:1–15.
6. Ross JS, Brand-Zawadzkii M, Moore KR. Diagnostic imaging, spine. Salt Lake City: Amirsys; 2007. p. I-1–152-154, II-2-48–59.
7. Arnoldi CC, Brodsky AE, Canchoix J. Lumbar spinal stenosis and nerve root entrapment syndromes. Definition and classification. Clin Orthop Relat Res. 1976;115:4–5.
8. Ullrich CG, Binet EF, Sanecki MG. Quantitative assessment of the lumbar spinal canal by computed tomography. Radiology. 1980;134:137–43.
9. Schönström N, Hansson T. Pressure changes following constriction of the cauda equine. An experimental study in situ. Spine (Phila Pa 1976). 1988;13(4):385–8.
10. Rothman SGL, Glenn WV, editors. Film organization and case reporting. Baltimore: University Park Press; 1985. p. 29–112.
11. Antonio L, Fabio M. Imaging del rachide: Il vecchio e il nuovo, vol. 3. Milano: Springer Verlag-Italia; 2008. p. 29–34, e37–39.

12. Sant-Luis LA. Lumbar spinal stenosis assessment with computed tomography and magnetic resonance imaging and myelography. Clin Orthop Relat Res. 2001;384:122–36.
13. Solarino M, Andreula C, Chiumarulo L. Malattia degenerativa del rachide. In: Faletti C, Masciocchi C, editors. Trattato di diagnostica per immagini nella patologia muscolo-scheletrica, vol. 2. 1st ed. Torino: UTET; 2005. p. 207–51.
14. Kang Y, Lee JW, Koh JH, Hur S, Kim SJ, Chai JW, Kang HS. MRI grading system for the cervical canal stenosis. AJR. 2011;197:134–40.
15. Muhle C, Metzner J, Weinert D, et al. Classification system based on kinematic MR imaging in cervical spondylitic myelopathy. AJNR. 1998;19:1763–71.
16. Stafira JS, Sonnad JR, Yuh WTC, et al. Qualitative assessment of cervical spinal stenosis: observer variability on TC and RM images. AJNR. 2003;24:766–9.
17. Meyer F, Börm W, Thomé C. Degenerative cervical spinal stenosis: current strategies in diagnosis and treatment. Dtsch Arztebl Int. 2008;105:366–72.
18. Elsing JPJ, Kaech DL. Dynamic imaging of the spine with an open upright MRI: present results and future prospective of FMRI. Eur J Orhopedics Surg Trac. 2007;17:119–24.
19. Greenspan A. Imaging in ortopedia: un approccio pratico, vol. IV. Roma: Cic Edizioni Internazionali; 2009. p. 397–9.
20. Bryk D, Rosenkranz W. True spondylolisthesis and pseudo-spondylolisthesis: the spinous process sign. J Can Assoc Radiol. 1969;20(1):53–6.
21. ACR-ASNR-SCBT. MR practice parameter for the performance of magnetic resonance imaging of the adult spine. Amended 2014, resolution 39.
22. Violaris K, Karakyriou M. Presentation of a rare case of bilateral lumbar synovial cysts. OJMN. 2012;2(2):25–7.
23. Epstein NE. Lumbar spinal synovial cysts: a review of diagnosis, surgical management and outcome assessment. J Spinal Disord Tech. 2004;17(4):1321–5.
24. Kelly BJ, Erickson BJ, et al. Compressive myelopathy mimicking transverse myelitis. Neurologist. 2010;16(2):120–2.

CT/X-Ray-Guided Technique in Lumbar Spinal Canal and Foramina Stenosis: Spacers

2

Giuseppe Bonaldi and Luigi Manfrè

2.1 Introduction to the Lumbar Spinal Canal Stenosis

The lumbar spinal stenosis (LSS) results from a narrowing of the spinal canal leading to compression of nerve roots contained in the dural sac and/or foramina. The LSS can be caused by many congenital (idiopathic or achondroplastic LSS), iatrogenic (typically post-laminectomy or post-fusion), and acquired conditions.

Narrowing of the spinal canal in *idiopathic* stenosis results from congenitally short pedicles; other morphologic features are thick, squat pedicles, trefoil-shaped aspect of the canal and lateral recesses in axial plane, and laterally directed laminae. Patients with this condition tend to become symptomatic later (beyond the fourth decade), frequently because of the superposition of acquired (although even mild) degenerative changes, which would be well tolerated otherwise. Other causes of spinal stenosis include excessive use of corticosteroids, either iatrogenic or endogenous (e.g., Cushing's syndrome), as well as Paget's disease and acromegaly.

Acquired LSS is by far the most common situation, and one of the most frequent reasons why a patient presents to a spine specialist [1]. The narrowing of canal and/or foramina is caused by a combination of a wide variety of age-related degenerative changes of the lumbar disks and facets joints: loss of disk height, bulging of the annulus fibrosus, ligamentum flavum infolding, facet osteoarthritis with hypertrophy and osteophyte formation, thickening of the joint capsule, and occasional synovial cysts. Facet hypertrophy and deformation often lead to degenerative spondylolisthesis, the primary level affected being L4–L5, followed by L3–L4.

Electronic supplementary material Supplementary material is available in the online version of this chapter at 10.1007/978-3-319-26270-3_2.

G. Bonaldi, M.D. (✉)
Department of Neuro Radiology, Papa Giovanni XXIII Hospital, Bergamo, Italy
e-mail: bbonaldi@yahoo.com

L. Manfrè, M.D.
Minimal Invasive Spine Therapy Department, AOE Cannizzaro, Catania, Italy

© Springer International Publishing Switzerland 2016
L. Manfrè (ed.), *Spinal Canal Stenosis*, New Procedures in Spinal Interventional Neuroradiology, DOI 10.1007/978-3-319-26270-3_2

Symptoms of nerve root compression in the dural sac or foramina are those of intermittent neurogenic claudication (INC) [2–4]: discomfort and pain radiating to buttocks, thigh, and lower limbs during standing and walking. Symptoms are exacerbated by lumbar extension and relieved by flexion. Patients do better sitting or biking, or they feel more comfortable going up rather than going down stairs or slopes. This happens because standing narrows the neural foramina and canal area resulting in impingement, whereas flexing (such as when sitting or riding a bike or walking uphill) enlarges the spinal canal area, relieving impingement. Physical examination may reveal a wide-based gait and unsteadiness, due to involvement of the proprioceptive fibers in the posterior columns [5]. A sensory or motor deficit occurs in about half of patients, and the deficit may occur bilaterally, frequently involving more than one specific nerve. Motor findings are typically mild, and functionally limiting lower limb weakness is uncommon [5].

Onset of symptoms, although not yet completely elucidated, seems related to pressure on the venules surrounding the nerve roots, leading to engorgement and ischemic nerve impairment [6–12]. Such ischemic mechanisms also accounts for immediate reversibility of symptoms as pressure on venules/nerve structures is relieved (i.e., patients stop walking or sit or bend their back forward), much like vascular claudication. This behavior of symptoms also explains the definition of claudication as intermittent.

Treatment of symptomatic LSS can be *conservative*, using medications, exercises and physiotherapy programs, and pain-controlling injections. The majority of symptomatic patients managed nonoperatively report no substantial change over the course of 1 year [13–15].

Operative treatment traditionally consists of decompression of the spinal canal with laminectomies and/or partial facet arthrectomy with or without instrumented stabilization. The last decades have seen a growing trend in use of minimally invasive techniques in spine surgery for the degenerated lumbar spine, which use smaller incisions with minimal soft tissue trauma and more limited removal of the laminae and facet joints, have a low rate of complications, significantly reducing the hospitalization, often on an outpatient basis. Minimally invasive surgical approaches and implants can be used to avoid or delay more aggressive procedures, and their use as "intermediate" solutions is justified as long as iatrogenic trauma during implantation is minimal.

Non-dynamic percutaneous spacers represent an even less invasive alternative to conventional open surgery for patients with mild/moderate LSS, who failed conservative treatments. Despite surgical indication for spacer introduction has been recently extended to lumbar discogenic pain, facet joint syndrome, disk herniation and low-grade instability, mild spinal canal stenosis remains the main disease to be treated with [16]. Moreover, percutaneous spacers are cheaper and safer than instrumented fusion procedures and do not preclude further therapeutic options. Thus, although many questions are yet to be answered and further studies are required to determine the optimal design of implants, such devices and surgical approaches may represent a valuable tool in the hands of not only spine surgeons but also of interventional radiologists.

2.2   Biomechanics of LSS and Spacers

The basic functional spinal unit (SU) is the smallest physiological unit of motion of the spine. It is therefore termed as "motion segment." It consists of two adjacent vertebrae, the disk and all the connecting ligaments. Individual motion segments contribute to the total motion of the spine. The components and movements of the SU are extremely complex, and the biomechanics of SUs are neither fully understood nor simple to explain.

Nevertheless, we will try to summarize the main concepts on which the designs of the different interspinous devices are based, be they used either for treatment of canal and foramina stenosis or as local stabilizers for treatment of back pain from moderate instability.

In flexion and extension, muscles apply a bending moment to the SU. The bending moment (M) corresponds to two vector forces applied in opposite directions with a distance between them different from 0 and is measured as a force (F) multiplied by a distance (d): $M=Fd$ (Fig. 2.1). During flexion of the lumbar spine, muscles apply a bending moment to the SUs. The total motion obtained (modification of posture from neutral to flexion) is the sum of the modifications obtained at the level of each single SU, i.e., a decrease of the anterior disk height and a widening of the posterior structures (particularly of the interspinous space), which are stretched and moved apart. The supraspinous ligament is the structure limiting flexion more effectively.

The opposite happens in extension, with an increase in the anterior disk height and closing of the interspinous space.

2.2.1   The Neutral Zone (NZ)

The NZ (Fig. 2.2) is the position of the SU in which a small bending moment can result in a large movement (i.e., a large change in the angles between the two vertebrae). In a normal SU, the center of the NZ corresponds to the middle position

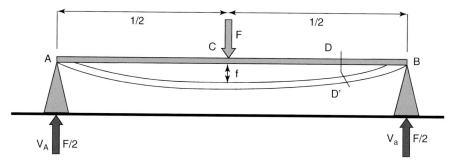

Fig. 2.1   A bending moment exists in a structural element when a moment is applied to the element so that the element bends. Moments and torques are measured as a force multiplied by a distance: $M=Fd$

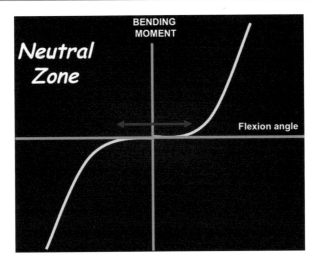

Fig. 2.2 Bending moment versus flexion angle of a SU. In the NZ, small differences in bending moment result in large changes of angle

between flexion and extension. A small moment is required to start flexion (or extension). However, with a progressive increase in the movement, it becomes increasingly harder to obtain new flexion (or extension). The NZ is a measure of the laxity of the SU, and it widens in the presence of instability. Pathological widening of the NZ allows exaggerated movements, which in turn require a large amount of energy for return to the neutral state. Dynamic devices, like the spacers used for treatment of the spinal stenosis, aim to reduce the NZ or to reposition it in the appropriate (nonpainful) place. A reduction of the NZ corresponds to a reduction of the local instability, and this in return corresponds to less irritation and compression of the roots traversing or exiting canal and foramina at the stenotic level.

2.2.2 Instantaneous Center of Rotation (ICR)

The ICR corresponds to the point at which, if a load is applied, no bending occurs. It is defined as "instantaneous" because it can change at every instant during different types of movements. As an example, think of a bicycle wheel. When the wheel turns round, the central pivot does not touch the ground; the ICR corresponds to the nonmoving center of the hub. However, in a moving bicycle, the only nonmoving part is the one touching the ground, and it changes at each instant (imagine the wheel turning as a whole around the fixed point in contact with the ground). Predicting the ICR in structures as complex as the SU is difficult. The ICR changes with different movements, and these changes become more unpredictable in the presence of instability. More often, in a healthy SU, in the standing, inactive position, the ICR is located posterior to the center of the disk (Fig. 2.3a), just above the inferior end plate [17] (corresponding approximately to the center of gravity).

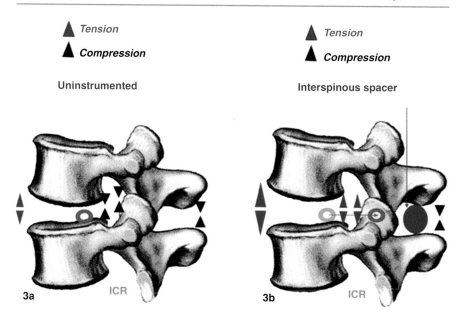

Fig. 2.3 The rigid interspinous spacer moves the ICR posteriorly (**3b**), modifying the loads on the different parts of the SU, in comparison to normal vertebral unit (**3a**)

It moves in flexion and extension, and the variability is considerable. There are no simple rules to predict the effect of stabilization devices on the ICR, but one is notable: the ICR moves toward an increase of stiffness.

2.2.3   Changes Occurring When an Interspinous Spacer Is Deployed

As the supraspinous process is preserved surgically when a spacer is introduced percutaneously, spacers do not modify SU biomechanics during flexion. During extension, the biomechanics are not modified until the spacer undergoes compression. At that moment, the ICR moves posteriorly behind the facets (i.e., toward the increase in stiffness determined by the device), thereby modifying the loads on the different parts of the SU (Fig. 2.3b). The reduction of the NZ and modification of the ICR given by the presence of the device totally modify the behavior of the SU and the loads in its components. The anterior annulus is stretched and an additional increase in the anterior height of the disk is obtained: the apposition of IS reduces disk load avoiding local anterior spinal column stress [18, 19]. To allow and compensate for this, the facets move opposite to the normal direction, opening instead of closing. That is, the amount of movement that is no longer obtainable at the expense of the interspinous space (decrease of the angle in extension) is now obtained at the level of different, elastic structures. An immediate consequence is widening of spinal canal and foramina, instead of conventional narrowing during the extension. Another consequence of spacer introduction is that the back pain induced in extension by pressure originating in the facets and/or posterior annulus may be partially relieved by unloading of these structures [20].

In a cadaveric study on the effects of an interspinous implants on disk pressures, Swanson and colleagues reported that the pressures of the posterior annulus and nucleus pulposus were reduced by 63 % and 41 %, respectively, during extension and by 38 % and 20 %, respectively, in the neutral, standing position [18] (Fig. 2.3b). Biomechanical studies have shown that the implant significantly reduces intradiscal pressure and facet load (Fig. 2.4a, b), as well as preventing narrowing of the spinal canal and neural foramens (Fig. 2.5a–e) [18, 20, 21].

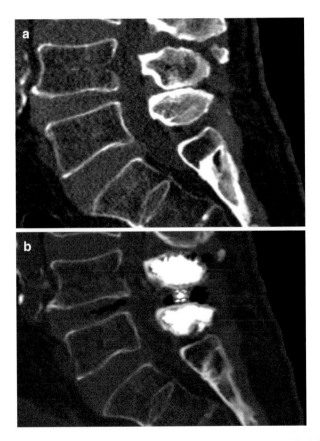

Fig. 2.4 Intradiscal pressure reduction after spacer implantation. On preop sagittal CT scan recon (**a**), marked lumbar sacral canal stenosis at the level of L4–L5 can be appreciated, with reduced interspinous space, interspinous ligaments bulging, and moderate local disk protrusion. After interspinous spacer introduction (**b**), there is an interspinous space and spinal canal widening, with the appearance of evident intradiscal degenerative gas, related to intradiscal pressure reduction. The spinous processes have been augmented with PMMA injection

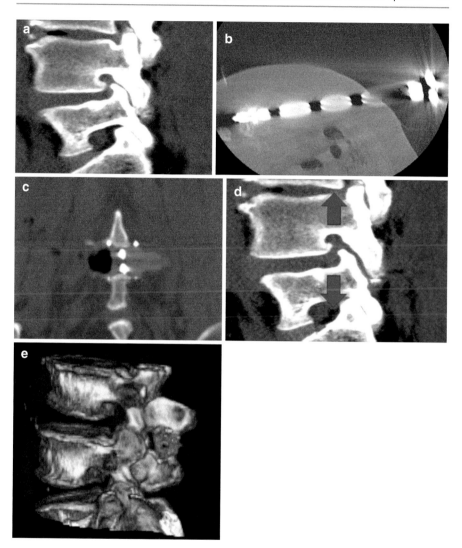

Fig. 2.5 Spinal foramina stenosis and spacers in a patient suffering from selective left L4 sciatalgia. On preop left parasagittal 2D CT scan recon, a severe narrowing of the left L4/L5 radicular foramina can be appreciated (**a**). A percutaneous spacer (Helifix®) is directly introduced via right paraspinal approach (**b**) using specific muscle dilator support. After removing the spacer dispenser, the device can be appreciated between the L4 and L5 spinous processes on a coronal 2D CT recon scan (**c**), widening in interspinous space. As a consequence of spacer introduction, left L4/L5 foramina is widened (*red arrows*), as appreciated on 2D (**d**) and 3D (**e**) CT scan reconstructions

In extension, the rigid interspinous implant significantly increases the canal area, subarticular diameter, canal diameter, and area/width of the foramen [18, 22, 23]. The final effect is that the implant prevents narrowing of the spinal canal and foramina in extension, thereby reducing or eliminating compression of the nerve roots.

2.3   Design Rationale of Devices for Treatment of Lumbar Stenosis and General Surgical Principles

There are two main categories of devices design: the *interspinous spacers* and the pedicle *screw-based* systems.

Rigid, non-deformable, non-dynamic interspinous spacers are the most widely diffuse ones for treatment of a stenotic condition, since they have a constant effect on the distraction of the spinous processes and consequently on the size of the canal and foramina. Low-rigidity, deformable devices (as pedicle *screw-based* systems) act more as shock absorbers, with a consequently more physiological action on range of motion of the SU together with an increase in bone compliance. They are more indicated for treatment of back pain generated by a local instability inside the SU/s (dynamic stabilization).

2.4   Interspinous Spacers

Originally, the interspinous process decompression system X-STOP (Medtronic) was proposed by Zucherman and colleagues [24] in the late 1990s for treatment of the symptoms of intermittent neurogenic claudication (INC) due to segmental spinal stenosis [2–4]. The X-STOP (Fig. 2.6) consists of an oval spacer positioned between the two spinous processes at the symptomatic level. The lateral wing is then attached to prevent the implant from migrating anteriorly or laterally out of position. The lamina and the intact supraspinous ligament also limit anterior migration and posterior migration, respectively. The central titanium-made pivot was rigid in the first version. Nowadays a PEEK layer covering the pivot makes it softer.

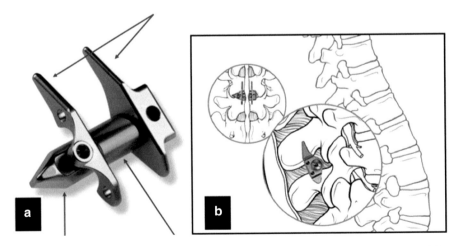

Fig. 2.6 In (**a**) an image of the X-STOP, depicting the lateral wings, the central spacer, and the tissue expander that pierces the interspinous ligament. In (**b**) the device deployed in the interspinous ligament, with the wings limiting lateral migration

It is deployed through a small posterior surgical approach. It is intended to prevent extension of the stenotic levels yet allowing flexion, axial rotation, and lateral bending [24]. Leaving the supraspinous ligament in place and intact has the double effect of preventing posterior migration of the device with no modification of the SU behavior when flexion occurs. Several different studies [18, 20, 21, 23–28, 40–42], including six cadaveric studies, report the effects of the device on biomechanical behavior of the lumbar spinal unit. Among them, the most important are limitation of range of motion in extension, increase in size of foramina and spinal canal, decreased loads in extension on posterior zygapophyseal joints, and decreased intradiscal pressure in neutral and extended position.

Similar percutaneous devices on the European market (still not yet approved in the USA) are available. Among them, in alphabetical order:

- Aperius (Medtronic)
- BacJac (Pioneer Surgical Technology)
- Flexus (Globus Medical)
- Falena (Mikai, Italy)
- Helifix (Alphatec)
- In-Space (Synthes)
- Prow (Non-Linear Technology Spine)
- Superion (VertiFlex)

But new devices are developed every day.

Superion and Aperius are rigid, being made of titanium, and are generally deployed through a percutaneous approach. BacJac, Flexus, Falena, Helifix, and In-Space are mainly made of polyetheretherketone (PEEK) totally or just in the area that came in contact with the lamina: PEEK is a semicrystalline thermoplastic that exhibits ideal strength, stiffness, resilience, and biocompatibility for spine surgery. It allows stress to be distributed more evenly on the surrounding bony structures, reducing an overload that could lead to acute fracture or chronic bone porosity and reabsorption. All of them are fully deployed percutaneously or through mini-open surgical accesses. The Prow is made of ultra-high-molecular-weight polyethylene (UHMWPE), a material used extensively for over 40 years in total joint replacements. Similar to PEEK, it has an elasticity modulus close to that of bone, granting support to adjacent bone with a lessened chance of subsidence.

Wallis (Abbott Spine) [29–31] and the DIAM (Medtronic) [32, 33] are double-action devices in which the interspinous spacer is secured with two tension bands wrapped around the upper and lower adjacent spinous processes. The bands also give support to the supraspinous ligament in limiting flexion of the SU (hence the double-action of the devices; more intense for Wallis and less for DIAM, whose surgical insertion does not entail sectioning of the supraspinous ligament). The Wallis is made of PEEK. The core of DIAM is made of silicone, whereas the outer mesh and tether are made of polyethylene terephthalate (polyester). Silicone is more resilient and compressible and is preloaded by compression before insertion. This permits posterior tensioning of the ligaments and disk, allowing a type of ligamentotaxis (particularly of the posterior annulus fibrosus). Biomechanical studies [19, 34, 35] showed the following data: decrease of both range of motion and intradiscal pressure at instrumented level with no significant change at adjacent level, and after discectomy, the angular motion was restored to below the level of the intact segment in flexion and extension but failed to stabilize in rotation.

Similar to DIAM is IntraSPINE (Cousin Biotech, France), which is made of the same silicone covered with a polyester textile. The silicone core has a shape based on a different concept compared with other interspinous devices. The central core fitting the interspinous space has an anterior part, designed to suit the interlaminar space. This kind of "nose," covered with a layer of silicone to avoid fibrosis in the yellow ligament area, gives the device a more anterior (ventral) point of action directly between the laminae, with a consequently more efficient action on the ICR (similar to that of the PercuDyn system, see ahead).

The Coflex (Paradigm Spine) is a U-shaped titanium device, inserted surgically between the spinous processes. This entails removal of all interspinous and supraspinous ligaments. Compared to dynamic devices, it is more rigid and, because of its shape, has more contact surface with bone. This could be an advantage over other interspinous/interlaminar decompression devices, thereby reducing the risk of delayed bone subsidence (see below in the "Complications" paragraph). Biomechanical studies [36–38] show that the device has a significant effect in reducing range of motion of the instrumented level, with no significant increase in range of motion at adjacent level when compared to posterior lumbar interbody fusion (PLIF).

2.5   Pedicle Screw-Based Systems

Screw-based posterior stabilization devices fall in a different category of design.

PercuDynTM (Interventional Spine) (Fig. 2.7) is a screw-based posterior stabilization device. Two screws are inserted with a totally percutaneous, fluoroscopy-guided approach through the pedicles into the vertebral body. The polycarbonate-urethane-resilient heads provide support to the inferior articular facets of the upper vertebra, thereby limiting their range of motion in extension. This device can be used even if a spinous process is not present (L5–S1 or postlaminectomy), a condition preventing the use of most of the spacers. Moreover, the device might have an effect even in treating true discogenic pain. The spacer is mounted more anteriorly with respect to a true interspinous device. Consequently, it exerts a more efficient action in moving the ICR outside the disk, forcing the segment into flexion into a neutral position and keeping the posterior annulus as distracted as possible. Thus, on a theoretical, biomechanical basis, it should decrease intradiscal pressure, reduce annular compression, and preserve posterior disk height in a more efficient way than more posteriorly applied devices [39].

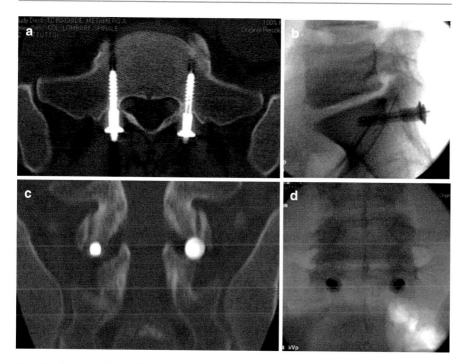

Fig. 2.7 The screw-based PercuDyn system. Titanium screws are anchored in the S1 pedicles *A*, while the polycarbonate-urethane heads of the screws support and cushion the inferior facet complex of the upper L5 metamer *B–C–D*, limiting its extension and unloading the disk

2.6   Clinical Evidence

Safety and effectiveness of the X-STOP device have been confirmed in a randomized controlled trial [24, 40, 41]. This prospective trial was conducted at nine centers in the USA. Two hundred patients were enrolled in the study and 191 were treated: 100 received the X-STOP and 91 received nonoperative therapy. Using the Zurich Claudication Questionnaire (ZCQ) criteria, at 6 weeks the success rate was 52 % for X-STOP patients and 10 % for non X-STOP patients. At 6 months, the success rates were 52 and 9 %, respectively, and at 1 year, 59 and 12 %. One of the most important results of the study is that the efficacy of interspinous device was proved to be comparable to previous reports for decompressive laminectomy but with considerably lower morbidity [24]. At 2 years, the mean improvement in the physical function domain was 44.3 % in the X-STOP group and -0.4 % in the control group. In the X-STOP group, 73.1 % patients were satisfied with their treatment compared with 35.9 % of control patients [37]. Results remained stable at an average of 4.2 years postoperative follow-up on 18 of the X-STOP patients [41] by ODI measurements; however only 18 out of 100 X-STOP-implanted patients were included in the study. These results were consistent with those reported by Lee et al. [42], although in a consecutive series of only ten patients. Other authors reported varying degrees of satisfactory outcome: 71 % at 1-year follow-up of 40 consecutive patients surgically treated with X-STOP implantation by Siddiqui et al. [43] and 31.1 % in the series of Brussee et al. [44]. Puzzilli et al. [45] compared in a prospective multicenter study 422 X-STOP implanted patients with 120 conservatively managed patients: at follow-up (with a minimum of 3 years) statistically significant improvements in the ZCQ and VAS scores were seen in patients treated with the X-STOP device but not in the nonoperative control patients at all postoperative intervals (P<0.05). During the first 3 years, in 38 out of the 120 control cases, a posterior decompression and/or spinal fixation was performed because of unsatisfactory results of the conservative therapy. In 24 of 422 patients, the interspinous device had to be removed, and the patients underwent open decompression.

In two recent randomized controlled multicenter trials, interspinous process device implant was compared to minimally invasive decompression [46] and to conventional surgical decompression [47]. Statistically significant clinical differences in effect between the methods were not found. Interspinous process device implanted patients had a higher risk of secondary surgery but lower complication rates.

Beyer et al. [48] compared in an open prospective non-randomized study of 45 patients the results of percutaneous interspinous stand-alone spacer Aperius with bilateral open microsurgical decompression: 5 patients out of 12 in the percutaneous group required implant removal and open decompression during follow-up.

In a multicenter randomized controlled trial in 391 patients [49], the Superion interspinous process spacer proved effective in relieving symptoms of intermittent neurogenic claudication secondary to moderate LSS in the majority of patients at 2-year follow-up. In this trial the controls were represented by X-STOP implanted patients: no clinical differences were seen between groups, and rates of complications and reoperations were also similar.

The Coflex device in addition to decompressive surgery was compared [50] to decompressive surgery alone in a total of 60 patients with lumbar spinal stenosis. At 1-year follow-up no statistically significant differences in outcomes were observed between the two groups, each consisting of 30 patients.

Wallis and DIAM were mostly used [51–55], rather than for treatment of pure spinal stenosis, with the aim to decrease range of motion at the instrumented level to treat mild segmental instability, to reduce intradiscal pressure and prevent recurrence of disk herniation at the same level, or to protect adjacent levels. The devices were used, in these studies, with a wide variety of lumber disorders and most of times in combination with decompressive surgery. All studies were also retrospective: consequently, no reliable conclusions can be drawn regarding their effectiveness in treatment of spinal stenosis.

In a meta-analysis [56] to evaluate the efficacy and safety of interspinous process distraction device (IPD) compared with open decompression surgery (ODS) in treating lumbar spinal stenosis, the authors found 21 publications, including 20 clinical trials and 54,138 patients. The results indicated that there was no significant difference in improvement rate, ODI score, and VAS scores of back pain or leg pain between IPD group and ODS group. The post operation complication rate, perioperative blood loss, hospitalization time, and operation time were lower/shorter in IPD group than ODS group. However, the reoperation rate in IPD group was higher than ODS group.

2.7   Contraindications and Complications

There are several contraindications to the use of interspinous implants (Table 2.1) [57–62]. Spacers induce segmental kyphosis of about 2°, minimally distorting the sagittal alignment, eventually leading to adjacent segment instability [61, 62]. Thus, a procedure involving more than two segments is not recommended (Fig. 2.8a–f). Interspinous spacers are ideal for treatment of L2–L3, L3–L4, and L4–L5 stenotic segments, even in case of previous different surgical procedures (Fig. 2.9a–f). The S1 vertebra usually lacks a spinous process large enough to provide a stable implant of the device: sometimes, however, thanks to a sufficiently large S1 spinous process, even the L5-S1 space is suitable for spacer implant, if the length of S1 spinous process is sufficient to sustain the spacer (Figs. 2.10a–d and 2.11a–e). The spine surgeon must consequently carefully evaluate such condition during the preoperative diagnostic workup [64, 65]. Only mild degrees of degenerative spondylolisthesis (grade I) are suitable for treatment with use of stand-alone interspinous spacers [62, 63, 66]: when facet joint mobility is maintained (viz., no significant degenerative articular block), spontaneous realignment of the grade I listhesis can be appreciated (Figs. 2.12a, b and 2.13a, b). On the contrary, conventional surgical stabilization/fusion should be considered in case of more severe symptomatic listhesis (up to grade II). True spondylolisthesis with isthmic lysis must be considered an absolute contraindication because the discontinuity of the posterior arch would not allow an effective segmental kyphosis [64, 66]. Scoliosis with a Cobb angle of more than 25° is correlated with poorer outcomes [64, 65, 67]. An osteoporotic condition must be considered to be a contraindication because of the risk of fractures consequent to the pressures generated against bony surfaces.

According to the literature, 3.8–11.9 % of patients treated with IS experience early recurrence of symptoms because of posterior laminae remodeling, generally

Table 2.1 Interspinous spacers: contraindications

1. Allergy to titanium or titanium alloys (or any component of the implant)
2. Spinal anatomy or disease that would prevent implantation of the device or cause the device to be unstable in situ, such as:
(a) Fracture
(b) Significant scoliosis with a Cobb angle >25°
(c) Degenerative spondylolisthesis greater than grade 1.0 on a scale of 1 to 4
(d) True spondylolisthesis due to isthmic lysis (because the action of the device would widen and aggravate the lysis and not modify the degree of the olysthesis)
3. Ankylosed segment at the affected level(s)
4. Cauda equina syndrome (defined as neural compression causing neurogenic dysfunction of the bowel or bladder)
5. Active systemic infection or infection localized to implantation site
6. A diagnosis of severe osteoporosis defined as bone mineral density (from dual energy X-ray absorptiometry or a comparable study) in the spine or hip that is >2.5 standard deviations below the mean of normal adult values

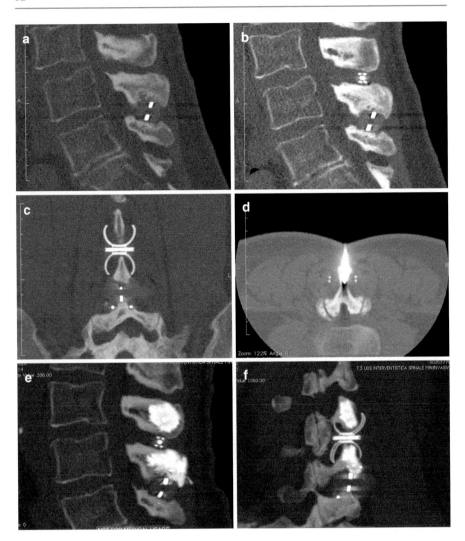

Fig. 2.8 Two contiguous spacer introduction in a patient with multilevel spinal canal stenosis. The patient was originally treated for selective L4/L5 lumbar spinal canal stenosis with a fully PEEK covered 12 mm spacer (Helifix®) with minimal lamina bone remodeling after 1 year (**a**). Because of recurrent spinal canal syndrome, he underwent MR scan demonstrating new LSC stenosis at L3/L4 level. A second 8 mm spacer (In-Space®) was introduced at that level, showed on sagittal (**b**) and coronal (**c**) 2D recon CT scans. Preventing further bone lamina remodeling, a small 12G Jamshidi needles were introduced into the L3 and L4 spinous process via sagittal route (**d**) and 1–2 cc of PMMA were injected (laminoplasty), protecting the spinous processes from future reabsorption or fracture (**e, f**)

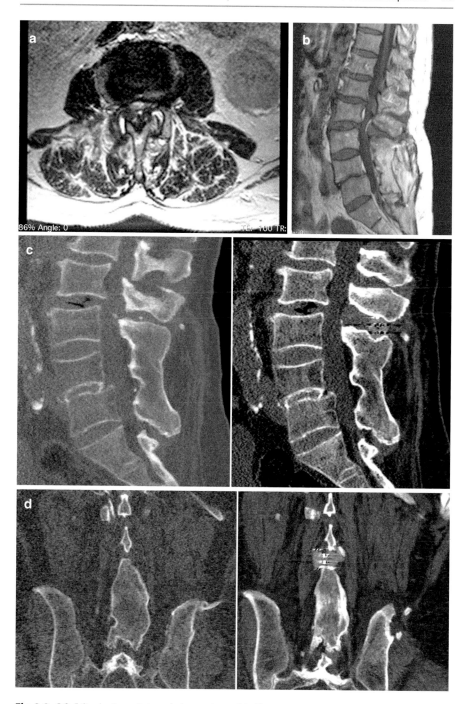

Fig. 2.9 L2–L3 spinal canal stenosis in a patient with 12 years previous L3 to L5 extensive surgical posterior fusion with bone graft. On axial (**a**) and sagittal (**b**) T1-weighted spin-echo scans, evident L2/L3 spinal canal stenosis related to ligaments bulging can be easily appreciated, just above the level of posterior fusion. After L2/L3 spacer introduction, widening of the spinal canal and interspinous space can be appreciated on sagittal (**c**, *right*) and coronal (**d**, *right*), in comparison to preop scans (**c**, **d**, *left*). 3D recons clearly depicts the correct position of the interspinous spacer (**e**, **f**)

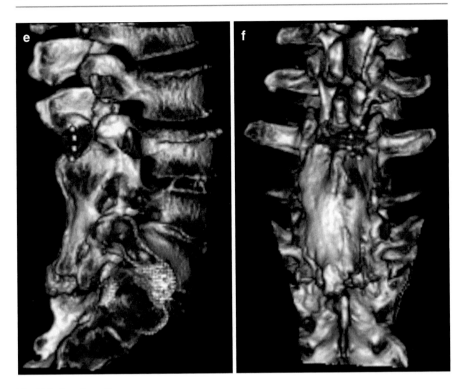

Fig. 2.9 (continued)

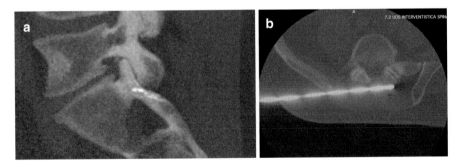

Fig. 2.10 Right L5/S1 foraminal stenosis in a patient with right L5 sciatalgia and L5/S1 stenosis. On preop 2D sagittal CT recon at the level of L5/S1 right foramina, evident stenosis of the foramen is detected (**a**). To reach the interspinous L5/S1 space, a guidewire is introduced in the patient pushing down the right hipbone; by doing so, the iliac crest is pushed down and there is enough space to introduce the straight guidewire directly into the L5/S1 space (**b**). A 10 mm spacer is introduced at L5/S1 interspinous space thanks to the sufficient length of S1 spinous process (**c**) and consequent widening of the radicular foramina is gained (**d**)

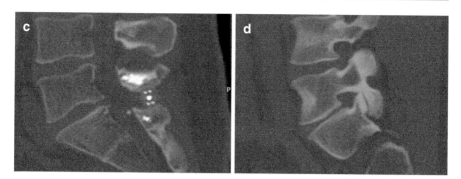

Fig. 2.10   (continued)

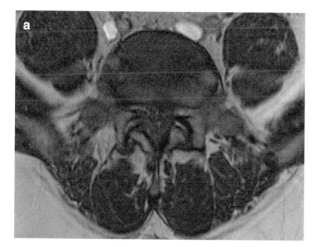

Fig. 2.11   L5/S1 lumbar canal stenosis and bilateral foramina stenosis. On axial (**a**) and sagittal (**b**) T1-weighted spin-echo scans, L5/S1 spinal canal as well as bilateral foramina stenosis is appreciated (more severe on the right side). Foramina stenosis is clearly demonstrated even on 2D sagittal and bilateral parasagittal CT scan recons (**c**). After L5/S1 10 mm spacer introduction and L5 and S1 spinoplasty, widening on the spinal canal as well as bilateral local neural foramina is clearly depicted (**d**), even on 3D image reconstruction (**e**)

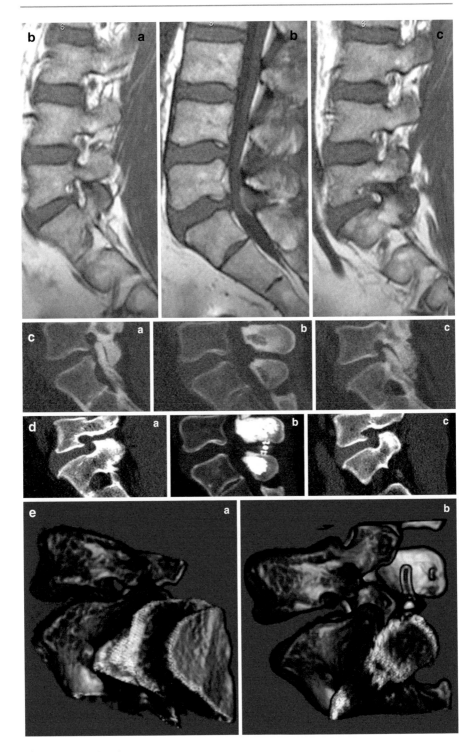

Fig. 2.11 (continued)

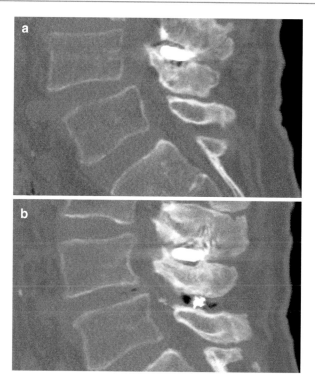

Fig. 2.12 Grade I anterolisthesis of L4 in a patient with recurrent spinal canal syndrome, L4/L5 spinal canal stenosis, and previous surgical introduction of a spacer at L3/L4 level. Prep sagittal 2D recon scan shows a previously introduced surgically spacer at L3/L4 level and mild anterolisthesis of L4, responsible for local LSC stenosis (**a**). After new percutaneous 8 mm spacer introduction, realignment of L4 to L5 can be appreciated, as well as widening of the lumbar spinal canal and interspinous process (**b**)

related to focal bone tenderness (i.e., osteoporotic disease and/or overload), reducing the distraction formerly obtained, even in patients treated with nonmetallic polyetheretherketone (PEEK) devices [68, 69], although most of the studies included less than 50 patients [62].

Barbagallo et al. [70] analyzed complications in a series of 69 patients. At a mean follow-up of 23 months, eight complications (11.5 %) were recorded: four device dislocations and four fractures of spinous processes. A prospective observational study found a high prevalence of fractures of spinous processes in 38 patients (50 implants) after implantation of interspinous stand-alone devices [71]. A fracture was not identifiable on plain radiographs, but postoperative computed tomography identified non-displaced spinous process factures in 11 patients (28.9 % of patients, 22 % of levels). Direct interview of patients as well as review of medical records indicated that five fractures were associated with mild-to-moderate lumbar back pain, and six fractures were asymptomatic. Three of the 11 patients underwent device removal and laminectomy for persistent pain. Fractures

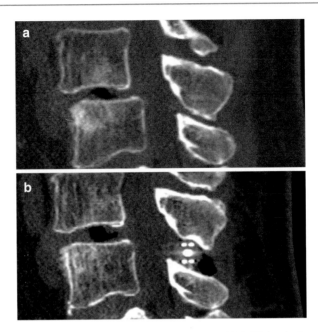

Fig. 2.13 Grade I anterolisthesis of L3 to L4 in a patient with L3/L4 spinal canal degenerative stenosis. On preop 2D CT sagittal recon scan, anterolisthesis grade I of L3 can be appreciated, with minimal intradiscal degenerative vacuum and bone sclerosis of the subchondral vertebral bone (**a**). After 12 mm spacer introduction, evident widening of the local lumbar spinal canal, as well as intervertebral disk space and realignment of L3 to L4 vertebra can be appreciated (**b**)

in the other three patients had healed by 1 year. A "sandwich phenomenon" fracture related to double X-STOP surgery was described also [72]. In a recent study [73], feasibility and efficacy of cement augmentation of the posterior vertebral arch (spinoplasty) before spacer implantation in preventing perioperative and post-implant fractures/remodeling of spinous processes was assessed. On a CT-guided technique, introducing a very small PMMA injection through a 13G Jamshidi needle introduced into the spine process along the median plane or adopting a parasagittal oblique route, reaching the crus of the laminae directly, can augment the posterior arch. By performing prophylactic posterior arch augmentation, one can reduce the failure of the percutaneous IS treatment, particularly in that patients. Spinoplasty seemed effective in preventing delayed fractures of the posterior arch after placement of interspinous spacers in patients at risk for fragility fractures. In some case, mild paraspinous leakage can be observed: as for conventional vertebroplasty, paravertebral leakage has not to be considered a real complication when asymptomatic [68, 74]. This is particularly true for the paraspinal area, were no main neural/vascular structures exist. Moreover, even in the case of patients who previously underwent spacer treatment with recurrent spinal

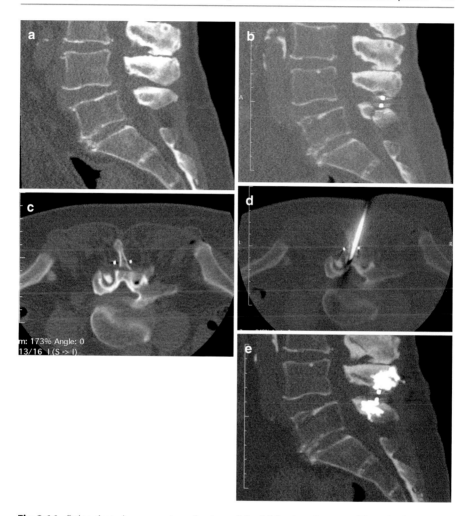

Fig. 2.14 Spinoplasty in spacer stress fracture of the L5 lamina. On preop 2D sagittal CT recon scan, severe L4/L5 spinal canal stenosis was detected (**a**) as well as on MR scans (not showed). Immediately after 10 mm interspinous spacer introduction at the level of L4/L5, a small fracture of the L5 spinous process was detected (**b**), the two parts of the spinous process lying on the sagittal plane (**c**). For this reason, a straight 13G Jamshidi needle was introduced through the fractured lamina (**d**) and fracture was instantaneously repaired by introducing intraspinous PMMA (spinoplasty) (**e**)

canal stenosis related to bone remodeling of the laminae, as well as patients with laminae fracture related to spacer apposition (Fig. 2.14a–e), a further treatment using spinoplasty and eventual new introduction of a second spacer at the same level can be performed, allowing resolution of spinal canal stenosis syndrome again (Figs. 2.15a–d and 2.16a–h) [75].

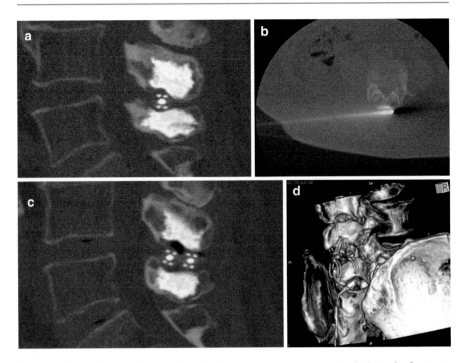

Fig. 2.15 Spinoplasty and double introduction of a second spacer posteriorly to the former at the same L4/L5 level, in a case of previous spacer failure related to bone remodeling. First, L4 and L5 spinoplasty was performed into the laminae, remodeled around the first original spacer (**a**). Then, a second straight K-wire was introduced percutaneously thanks to a CT guide, immediately posteriorly to the first spacer (**b**) and a second new spacer, posteriorly to the former is introduced (**c**), reopening the interspinous space: note the air bubble appearance above the former spacer after the introduction of the new one, related to the reopening. On a post-op 3D recon of the lumbar spine, the two spacers at the same L4/L5 level can be easily appreciated (**d**)

2.8   Spacers: CT-Guided Technique Description

2.8.1   CT-Guided Spacer Introduction

The treatment was performed in local anesthesia in a CT-room suite, using CT scan for introduction of K-wire in the selected interspinous space on a posterolateral approach, with a small 10–15 mm skin incision. C-arm was used for the introduction of progressive dilatators (from 8 to 14 mm according to the case), and final insertion of the maximal size of IS device was performed under fluoroscopic guidance. Total working time was 30 min approximately.

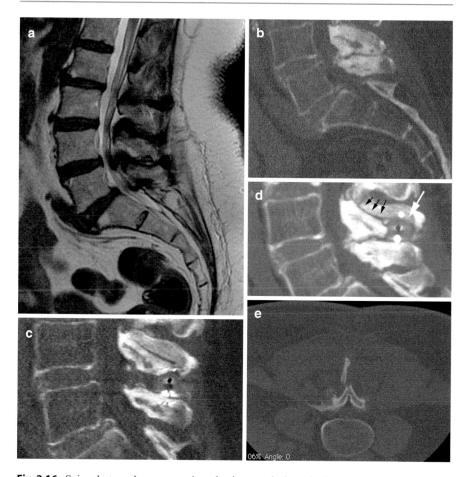

Fig. 2.16 Spinoplasty and new spacer introduction anteriorly to the former one, in a patient with L4/L5 degenerative spinal canal stenosis, and fracture + bone remodeling around the first spacer. On sagittal T1-weighted MR scan, severe L4/L5 spinal canal stenosis with bulging of interspinous ligaments was detected (**a**). 2D sagittal CT recon image shows extremely severe reduction of L4/L5 interspinous space (**b**), with apparent strong sclerosis of the laminae. Because of apparent spinous processes sclerosis, initial introduction of a 12 mm L4/L5 spacer was performed, temporally resolving the clinical signs of LSC stenosis syndrome (**c**). Nevertheless, after 8 months, the patient comes back complaining of new onset of similar clinical manifestation. On 2D sagittal recon follow-up CT scans, there is a large fracture of the L4 spinous process (black arrows in d) as well as complete remodeling around the first spacer (*white arrow* in **d**). The fracture fragments were none on the same plane (**e**): for this reason, a selective anterior fragment spinoplasty was performed, directly introducing a 12G Jamshidi spinal needle into the anterior part of the laminae (**f**), and complete spinoplasty of the area of the crus of laminae was obtained (**g**). Finally, reopening of the L4/L5 space was quickly obtained by introducing a second 8 mm spacer just anteriorly to the old first one, resolving the LSC stenosis syndrome pain related of the patient (**h**)

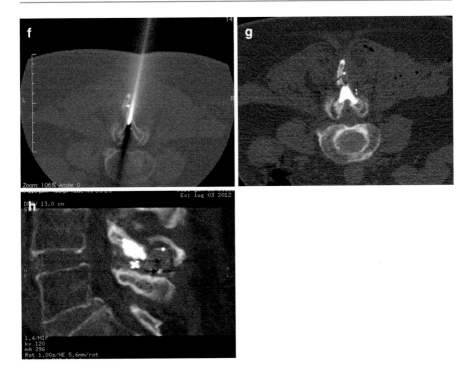

Fig. 2.16 (continued)

2.9   Spacer + Fusion

Spinal canal stenosis can be part of a more complex spine impairment including sagittalization of facets and spine instability, often creating the basis for ligament bulging and spinal canal stenosis. One of the drawbacks recently pointed out about spacers, is the fact that , although they are generally useful in widening the spinal canal as well as spinal foramina, they do not obtain fixation/fusion. Recently, new device have been created, with the double goal of obtaining widening of the spinal canal and fixation of the spinous processes. These devices include distal metallic wings, to be opened by the operator after being placed into interspinous space, engaging the distal lateral surface of the spinous processes, while proximal spiked end cap engages proximal lateral surface of the spinous processes. The system include the possibility to introduce inside bone filler, to accelerate fusion. By doing this, both spacing plus fusion can be obtained (Fig. 2.17).

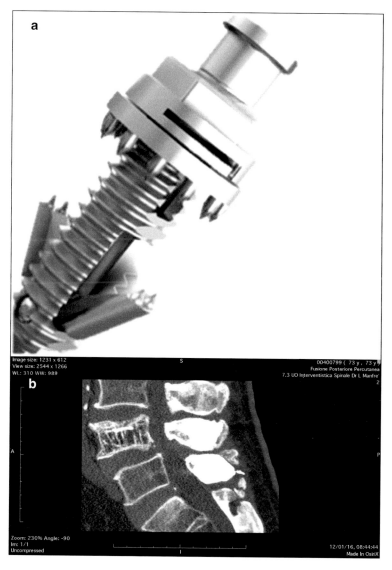

Fig. 2.17 Spacer & Fixation. The system consist of a spacer with distal opening wings and proximal spiked end cap, including holes to be filled with bone filler (**a**). After reinforcing the spinous process introducing PMMA, a technique called "spinoplasty" (**b**) the spacer is introduced through dedicated dilators (**c**) and when the final position is reached, fixation is obtained by spiked end round cap (**d**) and distal opening of two metallic wings (**e**)

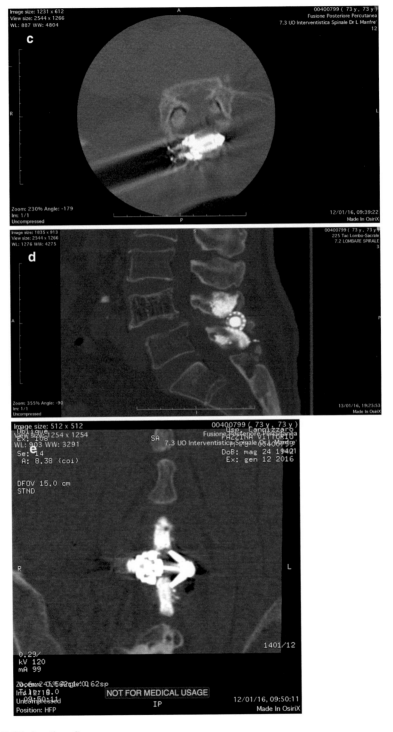

Fig. 2.17 (continued)

References

1. Deyo RA, Gray DT, Kreuter W, Mirza S, Martin BI. United States trends in lumbar fusion surgery for degenerative conditions. Spine. 2005;30(12):1441–5; discussion 1446–7.
2. Katz JN, Harris MB. Lumbar spinal stenosis. N Engl J Med. 2008;358:818–25.
3. Arbit E, Pannullo S. Lumbar stenosis: a clinical review. Clin Orthop. 2001;384:137–43.
4. Blau JN, Logue V. The natural history of intermittent claudication of the cauda equina. A long term follow-up study. Brain. 1978;101(2):211–22.
5. Katz JN, Dalgas M, Stucki G, et al. Degenerative lumbar spinal stenosis: diagnostic value of the history and physical examination. Arthritis Rheum. 1995;38:1236–41.
6. Jespersen SM, Hansen ES, Høy K, et al. Two-level spinal stenosis in minipigs: hemodynamic effects of exercise (1996). Spine. 1995;20:2765–73.
7. Porter RW. Spinal stenosis and neurogenic claudication. Spine. 2000;21:2046–52.
8. Takenobu Y, Katsube N, Marsala M, Kondo K. Model of neuropathic intermittent claudication in the rat: methodology and application. J Neurosci Methods. 2001;104:191–8.
9. Olmarker K, Holm S, Rosenqvist AL, Rydevik B. Experimental nerve root compression: a model of acute, graded compression of the porcine cauda equina and an analysis of neural and vascular anatomy. Spine. 1991;16:61–9.
10. Olmarker K, Rydevik B. Single- versus double-level nerve root compression: an experimental study on the porcine cauda equina with analyses of nerve impulse conduction properties. Clin Orthop Relat Res. 1992;279:35–9.
11. Olmarker K, Rydevik B, Holm S. Edema formation in spinal nerve roots induced by experimental, graded compression: an experimental study on the pig cauda equina with special reference to differences in effects between rapid and slow onset of compression. Spine. 1989;14:569–73.
12. Olmarker K, Rydevik B, Holm S, Bagge U. Effects of experimental graded compression on blood flow in spinal nerve roots: a vital microscopic study on the porcine cauda equina. J Orthop Res. 1989;7:817–23.
13. Atlas SJ, Keller RB, Robson D, Deyo RA, Singer DE. Surgical and nonsurgical management of lumbar spinal stenosis: four-year outcomes from the Maine Lumbar Spine Study. Spine. 2000;25:556–62.
14. Benoist M. The natural history of lumbar degenerative spinal stenosis. Joint Bone Spine. 2002;69:450–7.
15. Simotas AC, Dorey FJ, Hansraj KK, Cammisa Jr F. Nonoperative treatment for lumbar spinal stenosis: clinical and outcome results and a 3-year survivorship analysis. Spine. 2000;25:197–204.
16. Fabrizi A, et al. Interspinous spacers in the treatment of degenerative lumbar spinal disease: our experience with DIAM and Aperius devices. Eur Spine J. 2011;20 Suppl 1:S20–6.
17. McNally DS. Rationale for dynamic stabilization. In: Kim D, Cammisa FP, Fessler RG, editors. Dynamic reconstruction of the spine. New York: Thieme; 2006. p. 237–43.
18. Swanson KE, Lindsey DP, Hsu KY, Zucherman JF, Yerby SA. The effects of an interspinous implant on intervertebral disc pressures. Spine. 2003;28(1):26–32.
19. Bellini CM, Galbusera F, Raimondi MT, Mineo GV, Brayda- Bruno M. Biomechanics of the lumbar spine after dynamic stabilization. J Spinal Disord Tech. 2007;20(6):423–9.
20. Wiseman C, Lindsey DP, Fredrick AD, Yerby SA. The effect of an interspinous process implant on facet loading during extension. Spine. 2005;30:903–7.
21. Richards JC, Majumdar S, Lindsey DP, Beaupre GS, Yerby SA. The treatment mechanism of an interspinous process implant for lumbar neurogenic intermittent claudication. Spine. 2005;30:744–9.
22. Siddiqui M, Nicol M, Karadimas E, Smith F, Wardlaw D. The positional magnetic resonance imaging changes in the lumbar spine following insertion of a novel interspinous process distraction device. Spine. 2005;30:2677–82.
23. Siddiqui M, Karadimas E, Nicol M. Influence of X-Stop on neural foramina and spinal canal area in spinal stenosis. Spine. 2006;31:2958–62.

24. Zucherman JF, Hsu KY, Hartjen CA, Mehalic TF, Implicito DA, Martin MJ, et al. A prospective randomized multi-center study for the treatment of lumbar spinal stenosis with the X-Stop interspinous implant: 1-year results. Eur Spine J. 2004;13:22–31.
25. Lindsey DP, Swanson KE, Fuchs P, Hsu KY, Zucherman JF, Yerby SA. The effects of an interspinous implant on the kinematics of the instrumented and adjacent levels in the lumbar spine. Spine. 2003;28:2192–7.
26. Wilke HJ, Drumm J, Haussler K, et al. Biomechanical effect of different lumbar interspinous implants on flexibility and intradiscal pressure. Eur Spine J. 2008;17:1049–56.
27. Siddiqui M, Karadimas E, Nicol M, et al. Effects of X-Stop device on sagittal lumbar spine kinematics in spinal stenosis. J Spinal Disord Tech. 2006;19:328–33.
28. Fuchs PD, Lindsey DP, Hsu KY, et al. The use of an interspinous implant in conjunction with a graded facetectomy procedure. Spine. 2005;30:1266–72; discussion 73–4.
29. Sénégas J, Etchevers JP, Baulny D, Grenier F. Widening of the lumbar vertebral canal as an alternative to laminectomy, in the treatment of lumbar stenosis. Fr J Orthop Surg. 1988;2:93–9.
30. Sénégas J. Surgery of the intervertebral ligaments, alternative to arthrodesis in the treatment of degenerative instabilities. Acta Orthop Belg. 1991;57 Suppl 1:221–6 [In French].
31. Sénégas J. Mechanical supplementation by non-rigid fixation in degenerative intervertebral lumbar segments: the Wallis system. Eur Spine J. 2002;11 Suppl 2:164–9.
32. Taylor J. Nonfusion technologies of the posterior column: a new posterior shock absorber. In: Presented at the International Symposium on Intervertebral Disc Replacement and Non-Fusion Technology; 2001. p. 3–5.
33. Taylor J, Ritland S. Technical and anatomical considerations for the placement of a posterior interspinous stabilizer. In: Mayer HM, editor. Minimally invasive spine surgery. Berlin: Springer p; 2006. p. 466–75.
34. Lafage V, Gangnet N, Senegas J, et al. New interspinous implant evaluation using an in vitro biomechanical study combined with a finite-element analysis. Spine. 2007;32:1706–13.
35. Phillips FM, Voronov LI, Gaitanis IN, et al. Biomechanics of posterior dynamic stabilizing device (DIAM) after facetectomy and discectomy. Spine J. 2006;6:714–22.
36. Trautwein FT, Lowery GL, Wharton ND, et al. Determination of the in vivo posterior loading environment of the Coflex interlaminar-interspinous implant. Spine J. 2010;10:244–51.
37. Tsai KJ, Murakami H, Lowery GL, et al. A biomechanical evaluation of an interspinous device (Coflex) used to stabilize the lumbar spine. J Surg Orthop Adv. 2006;15:167–72.
38. Kong DS, Kim ES, Eoh W. One-year outcome evaluation after interspinous implantation for degenerative spinal stenosis with segmental instability. J Korean Med Sci. 2007;22:330–5.
39. Palmer S, Mahar A, Oka R, Gelalis I, Vraggalas V, Beris A. Biomechanical and radiographic analysis of a novel, minimally invasive, extension-limiting device for the lumbar spine. Neurosurg Focus. 2007;22:1–6.
40. Zucherman JF, Hsu KY, Hartjen CA, Mehalic TF, Implicito DA, Martin MJ, et al. A multi-center, prospective, randomized trial evaluating the X Stop interspinous process decompression system for the treatment of neurogenic intermittent claudication. Two-year follow-up results. Spine. 2005;30:1351–8.
41. Kondrashov DG, Hannibal M, Hsu KY, Zucherman JF. Interspinous process decompression with the X-Stop device for lumbar spinal stenosis. A 4-yearfollow-up study. J Spinal Disord Tech. 2006;19:323–7.
42. Lee J, Hida K, Seki T, Iwasaki Y, Minoru A. An interspinous process distractor (X Stop) for lumbar spinal stenosis in elderly patients: preliminary experiences in 10 consecutive cases. J Spinal Disord Tech. 2004;17(1):72–7; discussion 78.
43. Siddiqui M, Smith FW, Wardlaw D. One-year results of X Stop interspinous implant for the treatment of lumbar spinal stenosis. Spine. 2007;32(12):1345–8.
44. Brussee P, Hauth J, Donk RD, Verbeek AL, Bartels RH. Self-rated evaluation of outcome of the implantation of interspinous process distraction (X-Stop) for neurogenic claudication. Eur Spine J . 2007;17(2):200–3. Epub Oct 31.
45. Puzzilli F, Gazzeri R, Galarza M, Neroni M, Panagiotopoulos K, Bolognini A, Callovini G, Agrillo U, Alfieri A. Interspinous spacer decompression (X-Stop) for lumbar spinal stenosis

and degenerative disk disease: a multicenter study with a minimum 3-year follow-up. Clin Neurol Neurosurg. 2014;24:166–74.

46. Lønne G, Johnsen LG, Rossvoll I, Andresen H, Storheim K, Zwart JA, Nygaard O. Minimally invasive decompression versus X-Stop in lumbar spinal stenosis: a randomized controlled multicenter study. Spine. 2015;2:63–127, E61–132.

47. Moojen WA, Arts MP, Jacobs WC, van Zwet EW, van den Akker-van Marle ME, Koes BW, Vleggeert-Lankamp CL, Peul WC. Interspinous process device without bony decompression versus conventional surgical decompression for lumbar spinal stenosis: 2-year results of a double-blind randomized controlled tria. Eur Spine J. 2015;24(10):2295–305.

48. Beyer F, Yagdiran A, Neu P, Kaulhausen T, Eysel P, Sobottke R. Percutaneous interspinous spacer versus open decompression: a 2-year follow-up of clinical outcome and quality of life. Eur Spine J. 2013;22(9). Epub 27 Apr 2013.

49. Patel VV, Whang PG, Haley TR, Bradley WD, Nunley PD, Davis RP, Miller LE, Block JE, Geisler FH. Superioninterspinous process spacer for intermittent neurogenic claudication secondary to moderate lumbar spinal stenosis: two-year results from a randomized controlled FDA-IDE pivotal trial. Spine. Spine (Phila Pa 1976). 2015; 1;40(5):275–82.

50. Richter A, Schutz C, Hauck M, et al. Does an interspinous device (Coflex) improve the outcome of decompressive surgery in lumbar spinal stenosis? One-year follow up of a prospective case control study of 60 patients. Eur Spine J. 2010;19:283–9.

51. Senegas J, Vital JM, Pointillart V, et al. Clinical evaluation of a lumbar interspinous dynamic stabilization device (the Wallis system) with a 13-year mean follow-up. Neurosurg Rev. 2009;32:335–41.

52. Floman Y, Millgram MA, Smorgick Y, et al. Failure of the Wallis interspinous implant to lower the incidence of recurrent lumbar disc herniations in patients undergoing primary disc excision. J Spinal Disord Tech. 2007;20:337–41.

53. Mariottini A, Pieri S, Giachi S, et al. Preliminary results of a soft novel lumbar intervertebral prosthesis (DIAM) in the degenerative spinal pathology. Acta Neurochir Suppl. 2005;92:129–31.

54. Kim KA, McDonald M, Pik JH, et al. Dynamic intraspinous spacer technology for posterior stabilization: case-control study on the safety, sagittal angulation, and pain outcome at 1-year follow-up evaluation. Neurosurg Focus. 2007;22, E7.

55. Taylor J, Pupin P, Delajoux S, et al. Device for intervertebral assisted motion: technique and initial results. Neurosurg Focus. 2007;22, E6.

56. Hong P, Liu Y, Li H. Comparison of the efficacy and safety between interspinous process distraction device and open decompression surgery in treating lumbar spinal stenosis: a meta analysis. J Invest Surg. 2015;28(1):40–9.

57. Rolfe KW, Zucherman JF, Kondrashov DG, Hsu KY, Nosova E. Scoliosis and interspinous decompression with the X-Stop: prospective minimum 1-year outcomes in lumbar spinal stenosis. Spine J. 2010;10:972–8.

58. Tuschel A, Chavanne A, Eder C, Meissl M, Becker P, Ogon M. Implant survival analysis and failure modes of the X-Stop interspinous distraction device. Spine. 2013;38(21):1826–31.

59. Lo Jr TP, Salerno SS, Colohan ART. Interlaminar spacer: a review of its mechanism, application, and efficacy. World Neurosurg. 2010;74(6):617–26.

60. Bowers C, Amini A, Dailey AT, Schmidt MH. Dynamic interspinous process stabilization: review of complications associated with the X-Stop device. Neurosurg Focus. 2010;28(6), E8.

61. Epstein NE. A review of interspinous fusion devices: high complication, reoperation rates, and costs with poor outcomes. Surg Neurol Int. 2012;3:7.

62. Verhoof OJ, Bron JL, Wapstra FH, van Royen BJ. High failure rate of the interspinous distraction device (X-Stop) for the treatment of lumbar spinal stenosis caused by degenerative spondylolisthesis. Eur Spine J. 2008;17(2):188–92.

63. Anderson PA, Tribus CB, Kitchel SH. Treatment of neurogenic claudication by interspinous decompression: application of the X-Stop device in patients with lumbar degenerative spondylolisthesis. J Neurosurg Spine. 2006;4(6):463–71.

64. Siepe CJ, Heider F, Beisse R, Mayer HM, Korge A. Treatment of dynamic spinal canal stenosis with an interspinous spacer. [in German]. Oper Orthop Traumatol. 2010;22(5–6):524–35.

65. Lauryssen C. Appropriate selection of patients with lumbar spinal stenosis for interspinous process decompression with the X-Stop device. Neurosurg Focus. 2007;22(1), E5.
66. Kim DH, Shanti N, Tantorski ME, et al. Association between degenerative spondylolisthesis and spinous process fracture after interspinous process spacer surgery. Spine J. 2012;12(6):466–72.
67. Richolt JA, Rauschmann MA, Schmidt S. Interspinous spacers – technique of Coflex™ implantation. [in German]. Oper Orthop Traumatol. 2010;22(5–6):536–44.
68. Idler C, Zucherman JF, Yerby S, Hsu KY, Hannibal M, Kondrashov D. A novel technique of intra-spinous process injection of PMMA to augment the strength of an inter-spinous process device such as the X-stop. Spine. 2008;33(4):452–6.
69. Shabat S, Miller LE, Block JE, Gepstein R. Minimally invasive treatment of lumbar spinal stenosis with a novel interspinous spacer. Clin Interv Aging. 2011;6:227–33.
70. Barbagallo GM, Olindo G, Corbino L, Albanese V. Analysis of complications in patients treated with the X-Stop interspinous process decompression system: proposal for a novel anatomic scoring system for patient selection and review of the literature. Neurosurgery. 2009;65(1):111–9; discussion 119–20.
71. Kim DH, Tantorski M, Shaw J, Martha J, Li L, Shanti N, et al. Occult spinous process fractures associated with interspinous process spacers. Spine. 2011;36:E1080–5.
72. Barbagallo G, Corbino L, Olindo G, et al. The "Sandwich Phenomenon": a rare complication in adjacent, double-level X-Stop surgery. Spine. 2010;35(3):96–100.
73. Bonaldi G, Bertolini G, Marrocu A, Cianfoni A. Posterior vertebral arch cement augmentation (spinoplasty) to prevent fracture of spinous processes after inter-spinous spacer implant. Am J Neuroradiol. 2012;33:522–8.
74. Anselmetti GC, Bonaldi G, Carpeggiani P, Manfrè L, Masala S, Muto M. Vertebral augmentation: 7 years experience. Acta Neurochir Suppl. 2011;108:147–61.
75. Manfre' L. Posterior arch augmentation using PMMA (spinoplasty) before and after interspinous spacers treatment: preventing and solving the failure? Interv Neuroradiol. 2014;20:626–31.

X-Ray Guided Technique in Lumbar Spinal Canal Stenosis: MILD

3

John D. Barr, Bohdan W. Chopko, and Wade Wong

3.1 Lumbar Spinal Stenosis and Neurogenic Claudication: Incidence and Pathophysiology

Lumbar spinal stenosis (LSS) is a common degenerative disease of the lumbar spine that affects up to 8 % of the US population, particularly those over the age of 60 years [1–3]. If the stenosis is critically significant, neurogenic claudication can result from nerve root ischemia with the underlying causative theory being venous insufficiency as a result of venous constriction that becomes critically aggravated by exertion typically by standing a short time or walking a short distance.

The resulting symptoms typically manifest as painful aching particularly in the buttocks and thighs, but may extend distally down the lower extremities, and may be either unilaterally or bilaterally. The discomfort can be resolved by sitting down. The relief tends to occur more rapidly if the patient forward bends at the waist, and this is thought to be due to the stretching of the ligamentum flavum, thereby thinning the ligamentum flavum and resulting in decreased venous constriction. Patients frequently complain of balance problems, which are, in fact, problems of impaired proprioception due to sensory loss. Many patients with symptomatic LSS and neurogenic claudication may be recognized by their tendency to ambulate with their upper body forward bent over a walker or shopping cart (shopping cart sign).

J.D. Barr (✉)
Department of Radiology, University of Texas Southwestern Medical Center, Dallas, Texas, USA
e-mail: john.barr@utsouthwestern.edu

B.W. Chopko
Department of Neurosurgery, Stanford University, Stanford, California, USA
e-mail: bchopko@stanford.edu

W. Wong, D.O., F.A.C.R., F.A.O.C.R
Department of Radiology, University of California San Diego, San Diego, California, USA
e-mail: wadewongcott@ucsd.edu

© Springer International Publishing Switzerland 2016
L. Manfrè (ed.), *Spinal Canal Stenosis*, New Procedures in Spinal Interventional Neuroradiology, DOI 10.1007/978-3-319-26270-3_3

The most common etiology is age-related degenerative hypertrophy of the ligamentum flavum (46 %), spondylolisthesis with or without ligamentum flavum hypertrophy (24 %), disc protrusion or bulge with or without ligamentum flavum hypertrophy (22 %), and hyperostotic changes (11 %) [4].

Conventional definitive therapy for symptomatic LSS has been lumbar laminectomy, a procedure that may have negative consequences. Benz reported a complication rate of 40 % in patients over the age of 70 years who underwent decompressive laminectomy for LSS [5]. Katz reported the need to reoperate in 23 % of laminectomy patients with LSS and still found that 33 % still had residual symptoms [6]. Extensive bone resection may lead to spinal destabilization, and extensive muscle dissection may lead to denervation of paraspinal muscles, lack of muscular support, increased biomechanical instability, and ultimately failed back syndrome [7, 8].

3.2 The MILD Procedure: Overview

MILD can be used to treat symptomatic LSS when ligamentum flavum hypertrophy is the dominant, or at least significant, underlying cause. Patients with LSS caused primarily by severe listhesis or facet hypertrophy are generally not amenable to treatment with MILD. The objective of MILD is to debulk the ligamentum flavum with minimal soft tissue dissection and bone resection through the use of microinstruments, fluoroscopic guidance, and identification of the anterior safe boundary of ligamentum flavum dissection by establishment of an epidurogram. Bone and ligament sculpting tools are passed through a 5 mm diameter working cannula under fluoroscopic visualization. The instruments are designed with blunt surfaces facing to the dura to accentuate safety and make dural penetration difficult and unlikely (Fig. 3.1).

3.3 The MILD: Patient Selection

The MILD procedure is indicated for patients with symptomatically activity-limiting neurogenic claudication or radiculopathy from LSS significantly attributed to ligamentum flavum hypertrophy. The diagnosis of neurogenic claudication is made by history and physical exam. Patients with symptomatic neurogenic claudication will present with a history of increasing pain, cramping, burning, tingling, and/or fatigue in the lower back, the buttocks, thighs, and eventually lower legs upon standing for a short time (usually 10–15 min) or walking a short distance (often as short as 50–150 yards). Temporary relief of symptoms usually requires a rest period of sitting and bending forward at the waist or lying down. Many of these patients will report progressively worsening limitations with activities of daily living such as standing in front of the sink to brush their teeth, standing in a shower long enough to complete bathing, or walking to the mailbox. Many who are candidates for the MILD will also find the need to lean forward over the shopping cart or walker when they visit the supermarket.

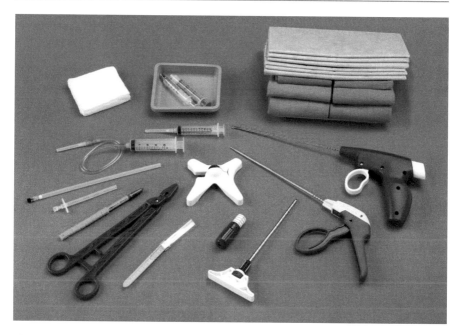

Fig. 3.1 Instruments used for the MILD procedure. From *right* to *left* are the tissue sculpturer, bone sculpturer, trocar-portal, depth guide, base stabilizer, #11 blade, forceps, marking pen, needles, and syringes

The physical exam should include documentation as to standing tolerance. A good way to examine this is to have the patient stand while taking the physical and measure the time for symptoms of neurogenic claudication to develop. A walking test can also be performed as further documentation.

The differential diagnosis includes diabetic or other neuropathy and vascular claudication. A significant fraction of patients, especially with an elderly population, may have elements of multiple disease processes. Consultation with neurologists or vascular surgeons may be useful, as well as electromyography (EMG) and vascular studies.

As these patients will often also have other features that may overlap with the symptoms of neurogenic claudication (e.g., sacroiliac joint dysfunction, greater trochanteric bursitis, lumbar radiculopathy), it is important to differentiate the various factors that may be contributing to the patient's total pain pattern. It is important to realize that neurogenic claudication resolves with rest, while many other pain etiologies remain persistent.

To confirm the diagnosis of ligamentum flavum hypertrophy as a cause of LSS, imaging preferably by MRI (alternatively by CT myelography) is used. Generally the finding of at least 4 mm of ligamentum flavum hypertrophy leading to at least moderately severe central canal stenosis is found. However the diagnosis of neurogenic claudication is formed on a clinical basis.

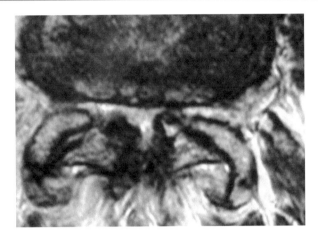

Fig. 3.2 A 87-year-old male complains of neurogenic claudication symptoms upon standing <8 min or walking <40 yds, requiring 15 min sitting for symptoms to resolve. MRI at L4–5 reveals right ligamentum flavum thickening of 7 mm and severe central canal stenosis

Candidates for the MILD procedure are those with symptomatic neurogenic claudication or, less frequently, radiculopathy from central canal stenosis caused by ligamentum flavum hypertrophy and who do not wish to elect to have a more extensive open surgical procedure or who are not considered to be good candidates for an open surgical procedure.

Poor surgical candidates would include patients with advanced age, comorbidities, and need for anticoagulation. Unlike some other open spinal surgeries such as discectomy, lumbar laminectomy with possible fusion is a highly invasive procedure with a prolonged and difficult recovery period (Fig. 3.2).

Contraindications to the MILD procedure include stenosis at a previous surgical site (due to postoperative scar or intervening bone fusion mass), stenosis at a highly unstable spinal segment, stenosis at a spinal segment not due to ligamentum flavum hypertrophy, underlying infection, unconsentable or noncompliant patient, and uncorrectable coagulopathy. Recent placement of a coronary stent or other device requiring maintenance of antiplatelet or anticoagulant drugs without interruption would also be contraindications to MILD.

3.4   The MILD Procedure: Preoperative Considerations

Once the patient is deemed a candidate for the MILD procedure, screening should be done to rule out underlying infection (e.g., elevated temperature, cellulitis) or any bleeding tendencies. If the patient is taking warfarin, that medication is typically discontinued 5 days prior to the procedure, and the patient may be transitioned in some cases to enoxaparin, which is then discontinued 12 h prior to procedure and an INR is obtained just prior to procedure. Patients on clopidogrel or any other antiplatelet medication are typically instructed to stop that medication 1 week prior to procedure. Even low-dose aspirin should be discontinued to reduce the probability of developing an epidural or other spinal column hematoma.

Informed consent should include a review of the indication for the procedure and a realistic discussion of expectations with the patient. The procedure and post-operative recovery should be explained in an understandable manner. Alternatives to the MILD procedure should be mentioned. While the serious complication rate for the MILD procedure is extremely low, potential risks (including bleeding, infection, allergic reaction, dural injury with CSF leak, spinal cord or nerve injury, paralysis, loss of bowel, bladder, and/or sexual function, and death) should be discussed.

Most MILD procedures are performed with local anesthetic and moderate conscious sedation (i.e., intravenous fentanyl and midazolam), so patients should be informed to arrive NPO 6 h prior to the procedure. As with most invasive procedures, most operators elect to administer a prophylactic antibiotic, such as two grams of intravenous cefazolin, immediately prior to the start of the procedure, so a review of patient allergies and adverse reactions is indicated.

3.5 The MILD Procedure: How Is It Performed in Detail?

First, any practitioner wishing to perform the MILD should undergo formal training and proctoring by the vendor (Vertos Medical, Aliso Viejo, CA). Prerequisite skills for the performance of MILD include proven experience and facility with fluoroscopically guided injection, biopsy, and/or interventional spinal procedures.

In starting the MILD procedure, it is important to properly position the patient in such a way as to best expose the interlaminar space(s) that will be accessed. As the procedure is performed with the patient in the prone position, the addition of a moderate bolster under the pelvis will help to introduce a degree of flexion of the lumbar spine. Also positioning the patient's arms along his/her sides will further help to accentuate flexion and widening of the lumbar interlaminar spaces (Fig. 3.3). However, avoid excessively severe accentuation of flexion as this can overstretch and cause thinning of the ligamentum flavum resulting in making removal more difficult.

Next establish surface paramedian guidelines between the spinous processes and medial borders of the pedicles as interlaminar decompression will occur along paramedian pathways over the lamina. Surface landmarks will help to avoid inadvertent excessive medial or lateral angulation of the instruments (Fig. 3.4).

The epidurogram is best performed at the operative level of the procedure. To keep the epidural needle out of the dissecting instrument's path, it is best to place the epidural needle in the midline at the superior aspect of the interlaminar space (Fig. 3.5a, b). The epidural space in MILD appropriate patients is frequently narrowed; the midline posterior-most aspect of the epidural space is often better preserved than the more lateral aspects. Alternatively, epidurograms can be obtained from points above or below the surgical site, but this usually necessitates using more contrast and potentially requires multiple injection sites.

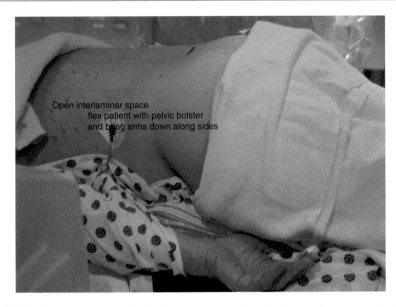

Fig. 3.3 Patients are positioned for the MILD procedure in a slightly flexed position using a pelvic bolster to increase the interlaminar distances

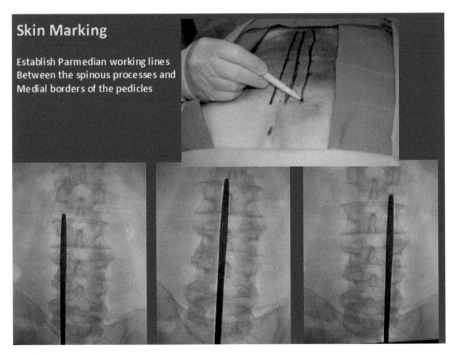

Fig. 3.4 Surface landmarks are drawn upon the patient's skin to delineate the midline and medial aspects of the pedicles

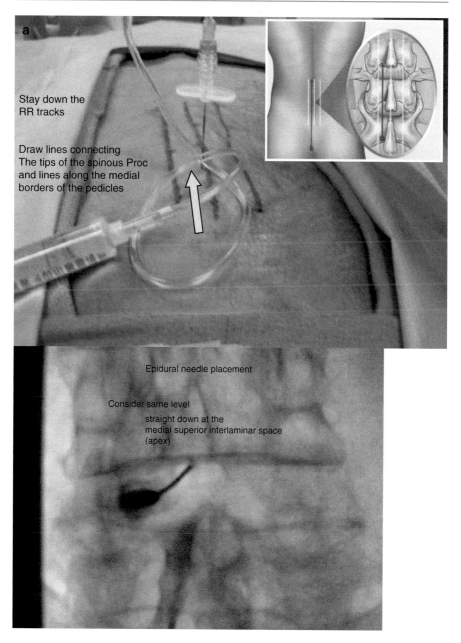

Fig. 3.5 (**a**, **b**) The epidural injection needle is inserted in the midline at the planned operative level (**a**). The fluoroscopic view shows the needle entering the superior aspect of the interlaminar space in the midline

Angulate the fluoroscope to the contralateral oblique approximately 45° to accentuate layering of the lamina. Pearl: align the adjacent superior articular process to bisect the posterior third of the respective disc. Place a forceps on the patient's skin along the ipsilateral drawn working parallel line to project its point in the direction of the roof of the lower lamina of the interlaminar space to be accessed (Fig. 3.6).

Confirm the trajectory by directing a long anesthetic needle along that intended course to the roof of the lower lamina (Fig. 3.7). Infuse the local anesthetic of choice to anesthetize the needle track from the skin down to the periosteum. Keep the needle in place as a guide for parallel placement of the access cannula system. The position of the long anesthetic needle should be critically assessed for the approach angle being neither too steep nor too shallow and for appropriate parallel and paramedian positioning. If the needle position is not precisely as desired, this should be repositioned and appropriate anesthetic injected before placement of the larger access system.

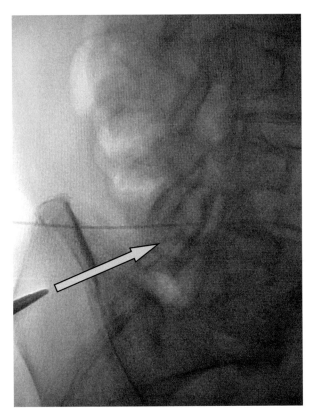

Fig. 3.6 The reverse oblique view shows the epidural needle in place with an epidurogram. The projected pathway of the planned entry delineated by the forceps on the patient's skin (*arrow*) shows appropriate entry position and angulation to reach the interlaminar space

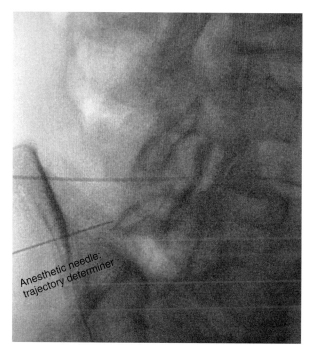

Fig. 3.7 The long anesthetic needle has been advanced to allow anesthetic infiltration along the pathway to the interlaminar space

If the anesthetic needle trajectory is satisfactory, this trajectory will then act as a guide for the trocar-portal. Make an incision with a #11 blade at the needle entry site and direct the trocar-portal in the same trajectory as the needle towards the posterior roof of the lower lamina (Fig. 3.8).

Attach the base stabilizer to the trocar-access portal and remove the trocar. Place the depth guide over the external end of the portal. It should be set at zero (Fig. 3.9).

Insert the bone sculpturer (Fig. 3.10a). Note that the bone sculpturer must be inverted in order to direct the cutting surface toward the superior margin of the inferior lamina. Most patients with symptomatic LSS have relatively narrow interlaminar spaces that prevent resection of the inferior margin of the superior lamina without first resecting part of the inferior lamina. Lay the sculpturer flat against the roof of the lower lamina (Fig. 3.10b), exert moderate positive pressure against the bone, and take a single bite using care not to release the laminotomy specimen until completely out of the body. Remove the extracted fragment, reinsert the bone sculpturer, and take another bite. The initial bites may feel softer because they consist of connective tissue on the surface of the lamina. The subsequent bites will feel harder and represent actual bone fragments. The extracted fragments should be retained for pathological analysis, as is typically performed upon tissue extracted during open surgical procedures.

Sufficient bone should be resected so that the bone sculpturer tool may be repositioned to allow resection of a portion of the inferior aspect of the superior lamina. The

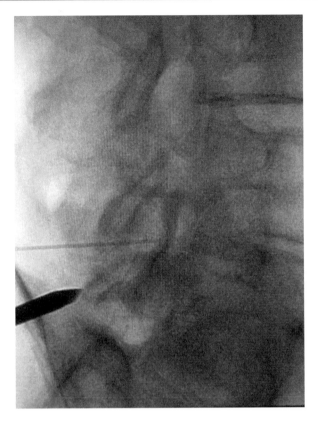

Fig. 3.8 The trocar-access portal has been advanced to the posterior/inferior margin of the inter-laminar space

bone sculpturer should be angled slightly in both the medial and lateral directions to facilitate resection of a wider portion of the lamina to maximize resection of the underlying ligamentum flavum. The medial and lateral extension of the initial access should extend only slightly such that the width of the lamina partially resected is approximately twice the diameter of the access portal. Referencing the parallel skin surface lines marked will help to prevent excessive angulation.

Pearl: It may also be useful to have a cadaveric or model lumbar spine available in the operating suite for comparison with the reverse oblique view, as this is not a typical radiographic projection with which the physician will have prior experience.

Rotate the bone sculpturer to access the inferior margin of the superior lamina (Fig. 3.10c). Apply moderate pressure against the bone and take a series of three to four single bites removing bone and ligamentum flavum through the portal after each bite. Slight lateral and medial angulation to extend the width of the resection should be performed, as with the superior surface of the inferior lamina.

Insert the tissue sculpturer (Fig. 3.11) after a sufficient laminotomy has been achieved to easily pass the tissue sculpturer past the laminae and into the ligamentum flavum. If there is difficulty passing the tissue sculpturer, return to work with

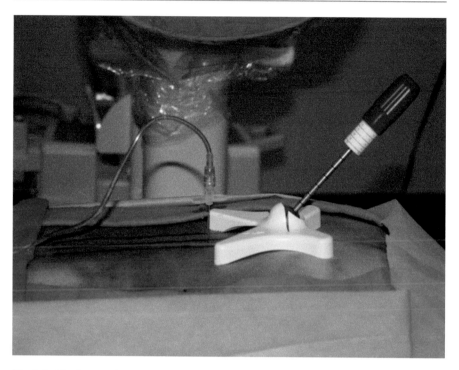

Fig. 3.9 The base stabilizer has been placed around the access portal to prevent inadvertent motion. The depth guide has been placed on the proximal end of the access portal; the depth guide should initially be set to zero

the bone sculpturer and perform a further laminotomy to widen the access. The tissue sculpturer should be passed initially at steep angle and then flattened to a more shallow angle as it is pushed forward in order to cause the jaws to open.

Unlike the bone sculpturer, the tissue sculpturer is not designed to be used in an inverted manner. The tissue sculpturer should not be tilted more than 30° off the vertical axis; otherwise it may project a sharp point toward the dura. The tissue sculpture has the capacity to gather three bites of ligamentum flavum tissue before it has to be removed from the portal and its specimen ejected.

Caution: Ongoing (live, continuous) fluoroscopic visualization of the interlaminar working space and epidurogram are vital to safe performance of the MILD procedure. The fluoroscopy mode may be changed to a low-dose, low-frame rate technique to help minimize radiation exposure to the physician and patient. The epidurogram should be refreshed with additional intrathecally approved contrast as needed. At no time should any of the instruments be allowed to cross deep to the epidurogram.

Caution: The safety of the MILD procedure relies upon proper visualization of the epidurogram, bony landmarks, and instruments. The procedure should be halted if adequate visualization cannot be obtained or maintained throughout the procedure.

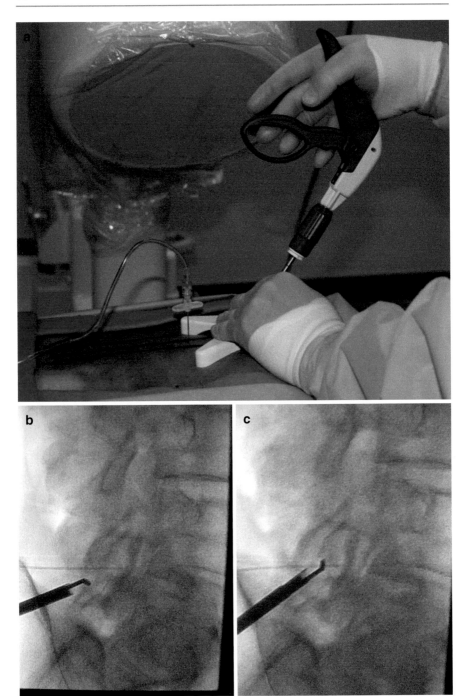

Fig. 3.10 (**a–c**) The bone sculpturer is inserted through the trocar in an inverted manner in order to resect a portion of the superior margin of the inferior lamina (**a**). The radiographic image shows the bone sculpturer on the surface of the inferior lamina; this will be advanced and then rotated in a caudal direction in order to resect the superior margin of the lamina (**b**). After the inferior lamina has been partially resected, the bone sculpturer is rotated into an upright orientation to engage the inferior margin of the superior lamina (**c**)

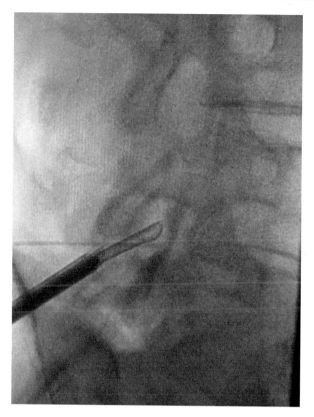

Fig. 3.11 After an adequate portion of the laminae has been removed, the tissue sculpturer is inserted to resect the underlying ligamentum flavum. Note that the tissue sculpturer is safely positioned posteriorly to the margin of the epidural space delineated by the epidurogram

Pearl: While viewing the fluoroscopic image in the contralateral oblique, frequently pay attention to the direction of the instruments along the drawn paramedian working lines on the skin surface. Often if there is difficulty in passing instruments to the correct depth, this is due to directing either too laterally (i.e., contacting the facet) or medially (i.e., contacting the spinous process) off the paramedian course.

Procedure endpoint: The goal of the procedure is to resect as much of the hypertrophic ligamentum flavum as is safely possible. When retrieval of ligamentum flavum fragments begins to yield only very small specimens with each bite, refresh the epidurogram. Upon visualizing an expansion of the epidurogram as in Fig. 3.12 (relaxation of the amount of thickening of the ligament), it is time to consider the procedure completed on that side. At times, the epidurogram may become less distinct with contrast leaking into the surgical bed so that definite expansion of the epidural space is not clearly demonstrated. This appearance, in conjunction with a paucity of ligament fragments being resected with each bite of the tissue sculptor, also represents a procedural end point.

At termination of the MILD procedure, the instruments should be withdrawn as a unit. They can be used for the contralateral side if a bilateral procedure is planned. Upon removal of the instruments, apply a few minutes of direct pressure over the

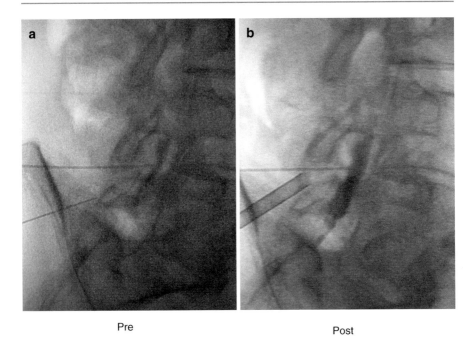

Pre   Post

Fig. 3.12 (**a**, **b**) Note marked change in the epidurogram pre- (**a**) and post- (**b**) MILD procedure. The expansion of the epidurogram correlates with debulking of the ligamentum flavum. Clinically this 87-year-old male progressed from standing tolerance of less than 5 min to unlimited standing and from being homebound to being able to walk at the shopping mall and resume active social activities after the MILD procedure

surgical site for hemostasis. At final termination of the procedure, Steri-Strips are used to close the small incisions and appropriate covering sterile dressings are applied. Suture closure of the small access incision is unnecessary.

Most commonly, patients present with bilateral symptoms and relatively bilaterally symmetrical LSS, such that bilateral MILD procedures are performed at a single level. Some patients may, however, have LSS at multiple levels amenable to treatment with the MILD technique. Other patients may have predominantly unilateral symptoms and asymmetrical LSS, typically those patients presenting with a significant radiculopathy.

The performance of multiple level MILD procedures presents some unique challenges. Until the physician has gained experience with the MILD technique, multiple level, bilateral procedures should be avoided. The reasons for the recommendation follow: even when refreshed with additional contrast, the epidurogram tends to degrade with increasing time, yielding a progressively more poorly defined demarcation of the safe zone for ligament resection. Patient discomfort and motion become more problematic with extended procedures. The cumulative dose of local anesthetic agents cannot be increased without limit. The use of general anesthesia to circumvent these issues is not recommended, as the safety afforded by the patient's intact sensation would be lost. Multiple level and bilateral procedures should only be attempted after the physician has gained the expertise required to perform MILD quickly and efficiently.

Tip: Although it may appear to be expedient to perform a two level MILD procedure through a single skin incision, the angle of approach to the second level treated will be suboptimal. Making a separate incision in the correct location will, in fact, result in a more efficient procedure.

Tip: Calculate and do not exceed the maximum recommended doses of local anesthetic agents. Be aware that any drugs injected may enter either or both the epidural and subarachnoid spaces.

The patient is sent to the recovery area and monitored postoperatively until returning to baseline mental and physical status. Expect to discharge typically in about 2 h post procedure. Instructions for follow-up and postoperative wound care are given to the patient. Postoperative medications should include an oral opiate for severe pain and acetaminophen or a nonsteroidal anti-inflammatory drug for mild or moderate pain. An antinausea medication such as ondansetron may be appropriate as well. Postoperative antibiotics are not necessary. Patients should not be discharged without supportive assistance continuously available for the next 12–24 h. Patients should be advised that they will probably experience moderate pain at the operative site for the next 2–3 days and that severe pain, fever, chills, or new neurological deficit should be reported to their physician immediately.

3.6   Postoperative Follow-Up

Generally a phone call in 24 h post procedure and an office visit at 1 week will be appropriate. At the 1-week post procedure visit, assessment can be made to assess improvements in standing tolerance and walking distance as well as Oswestry Disability Index. Wound healing can also be assessed at that time. In addition this is a good opportunity to assess for any other coexisting problems that the patient may have that may be contributing to the total pain profile, such as underlying greater trochanteric bursitis, lumbar facet disease, or sacroiliac joint dysfunction. As MILD patients tend to continue to improve as they regain strength and coordination after the procedure, a delayed follow-up perhaps at 6 months or a year may be elected.

3.7   Pitfalls and Pearls

3.7.1   Pitfall 1

An 80-year-old male complains of severe bilateral buttock and thigh pain upon standing for less than 12 min or walking less than 40 yards. His symptoms resolve after resting in the sitting position for about 20 min. You would like to obtain an MRI, but he has a cardiac pacemaker (pitfall). So you instead order a CT myelogram (pearl). The myelogram reveals severe stenosis at L3–4 and L4–5 and grade 2 spondylolisthesis at L4–5 (Fig. 3.13a). The neuroradiologist performing the myelogram then performs flexion-extension lateral views (pearl) to assess stability (Fig. 3.13b, c). The flexion-extension views demonstrate significant abnormal movement of L4 relative to L5, confirming an unstable situation. If unstable, a

Stenosis & anterolesthethesis

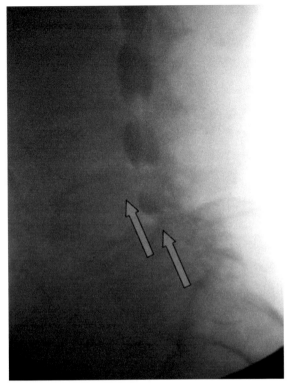

Extension   Flexion

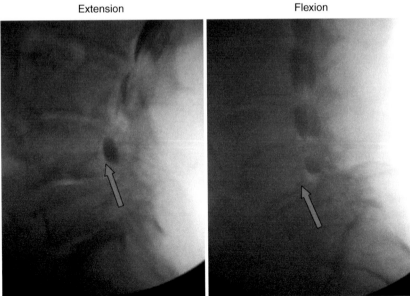

Fig. 3.13 (**a–c**). The initial lateral myelogram image shows severe concentric spinal stenosis at L3–4 and L4–5 as well as grade 2 spondylolisthesis at L4–5 (**a**). Sagittal T2-weighted lumbar spine MRI shows grade 2 spondylolisthesis at L4–5 (**a**). Extension (**b**) and flexion (**c**) images confirm significant instability at the L4–5 level

MILD procedure may fail to appropriately decompress the stenosis. Therefore, a surgical consult should be considered prior to offering a MILD procedure (pearl).

3.7.2 Pitfall 2

When setting up the bone sculpturer, a common mistake that beginning operators make is failing to protrude the bone sculpture beyond the portal. If the sculpturer is not exposed beyond the portal, a specimen will be prevented from being obtained. To obtain an efficient, substantial specimen, make sure that the bone sculpturer is well extended and firm contact is made against the bone surface (Fig. 3.14). Take your time when setting this up. Take a deliberate single bite, and remove the specimen by withdrawing the sculpturer completely out of the portal being careful to avoid losing the specimen in the patient or in the portal.

To collect a substantial specimen of ligamentum flavum, insert the tissue sculpturer like an ice cream scooper: first steeply downward then flattening out at a shallow scooping angle. This will help to accentuate jaw opening (Fig. 3.15).

Also remember that the tissue sculpturer is designed to be used in an upright (no more than 30° to either side of vertical) position. Otherwise the sharp upper shaft of the tissue sculpturer could be exposed to the dura as a sharp point.

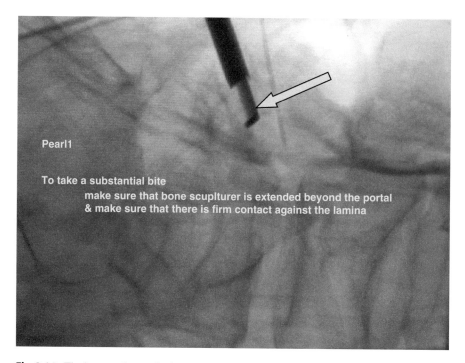

Fig. 3.14 The bone sculpturer is shown extending beyond the access portal so that the jaws may engage the lamina

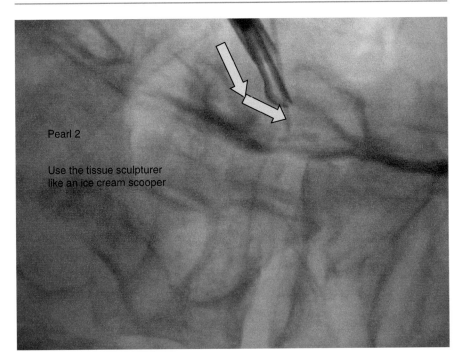

Pearl 2

Use the tissue sculpturer
like an ice cream scooper

Fig. 3.15 The tissue sculpturer is shown entering the posterior aspect of the ligamentum flavum at a slightly steeper angle that will be lessened as it is inserted more deeply

3.7.3   Pitfall 3

If the tissue sculpture is not flattened out, the upper jaw may be forced to close by tissue pressure and a substantial bite may be prevented (Fig. 3.16).

3.7.4   Pearl 3

To correct this restart with a series of shallower bites rather than trying to dive deeply too soon.

With your nondominant hand, grasp the shaft of the portal (Fig. 3.17). This will help to deliver pressure to the bone when performing the laminotomy and will help to control and coordinate fine movements of the tissue sculpture when decompressing the ligamentum flavum. It can also serve as a safety détente.

To be successful with the MILD procedure, it is essential to establish the correct diagnosis. It is possible for a patient to carry more than one diagnosis as exemplified by this 81-year-old male who presented with a history and physical findings consistent with neurogenic claudication and a right L5 radiculopathy from a combination of a right L4–5 synovial cyst and bilateral (left > right) ligamentum flavum hypertrophy (Fig. 3.18). This patient benefited temporarily from a right L4–5 transforaminal

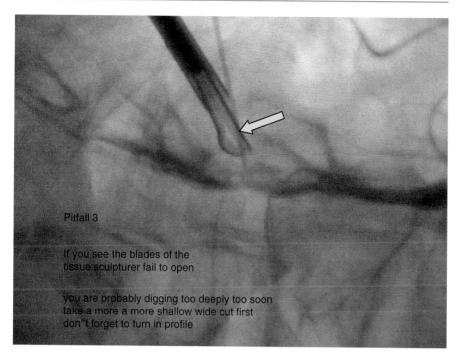

Pitfall 3

If you see the blades of the
tissue sculpturer fail to open

you are probably digging too deeply too soon
take a more a more shallow wide cut first
don"t forget to turn in profile

Fig. 3.16 The tissue sculpturer has been inserted at an excessively steep angle that prevented full opening of the jaws

epidural steroid injection and ultimately from a CT-guided decompression of the synovial cyst. However, the neurogenic claudication persisted until a MILD procedure was performed at L4–5. The sometimes confusing and similar clinical features of neurogenic claudication, radiculopathy, vascular claudication and peripheral neuropathy are summarized in Figs. 3.19, 3.20 and 3.21.

3.8   Treatment Options for Lumbar Spinal Stenosis

Treatment options for symptomatic lumbar spinal stenosis are relatively few. Decompressive laminectomy either with or without posterior spinal fusion has been the traditional definitive therapy offered. Whether or not this was superior to nonoperative therapies was evaluated in the Spine Patients Outcomes Research Trial (SPORT) [9]. Although a detailed analysis of the results of this trial is beyond the scope of this chapter, the results of the "as treated" group support a modest benefit for surgery vs. non-operative therapy. In addition, the relatively high crossover rate from non-operative therapy to surgery suggests significant patient dissatisfaction with traditional non-operative therapies. The disadvantages of lumbar laminectomy and possible fusion include the cost of the procedure as well as the prolonged and painful recovery period. Many elderly patients with LSS are simply too frail to

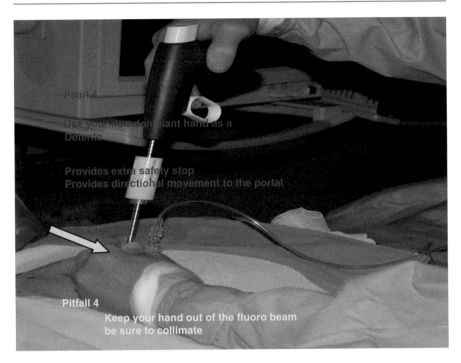

Fig. 3.17 The operator's nondominant hand is used to stabilize the access portal and to prevent inadvertent excessively deep tool insertion. Care must be taken to prevent the operator's hand from direct radiation exposure

undergo such a procedure, which has generated significant interest in less invasive alternatives. A variety of minimally invasive intervertebral implantable devices designed to increase the disc space height and/or induce mild forward flexion to increase the spinal canal cross sectional area have been developed. The only such device approved for sale in the United States, the X-Stop® Spacer (Medtronic, Minneapolis MN), has not proven to be a highly successful in clinical use. Burnett et al. performed a literature review and cost analysis of patients treated with non-operative care, laminectomy and X-stop [10]. They concluded that laminectomy was the most cost-effective choice. Patil et al. compared treatment with laminectomy to X-stop in a data base analysis and also concluded that laminectomy was the most cost-effective treatment [11]. Other interspinous devices available elsewhere may, however, eventually prove to be effective.

Although spinal cord stimulators have proved effective for a variety of pain syndromes, they do not usually benefit the symptoms of neurogenic claudication. They may be useful in the small subset of patients with LSS and predominant complaints of radiculopathy. Epidural steroid/analgesic injections may provide some temporary relief; as with spinal cord stimulators, relief is usually more significant for patients

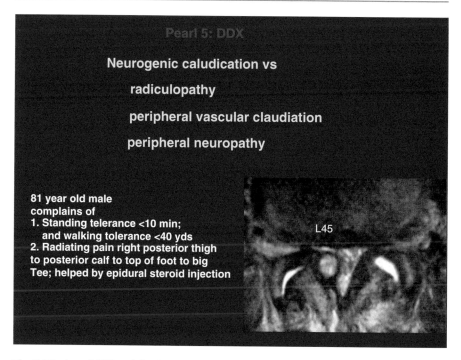

Fig. 3.18 An axial T2-weighted MRI shows a prominent right L4–5 synovial cyst in addition to bilateral ligamentum flavum hypertrophy. The patient had radiculopathy that improved after CT-guided decompression of the cyst and neurogenic claudication that improved after subsequent bilateral MILD procedure

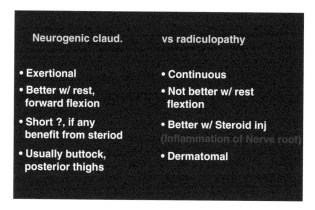

Fig. 3.19 The characteristics of neurogenic claudication vs. radiculopathy. Characteristics of neurogenic claudication vs. peripheral vascular claudication

Differentiating neurogenic and vascular claudication		
Activity/finding	Neurogenic claudication – symptoms?	Vascular claudication – symptoms?
Walking	Yes – relieved by flexion	Yes – relieved by stopping
Standing erect	Yes – relieved by flexion	No – activity driven
Bikingin flexed position	No	Yes – relieved by stopping
Peripheral pulse diminished	No	Yes

Note:
1. LSS patients compensate for symptoms by flexing forward,slowing their gait, leaning onto objects (e.g.,over a shopping cart) and limiting distance of ambulation.
2. Walking is worse in neurogenic claudication going downhill and worse in vascular claudication going uphill.

Fig. 3.20 The characteristics of neurogenic claudication vs. peripheral vascular claudication

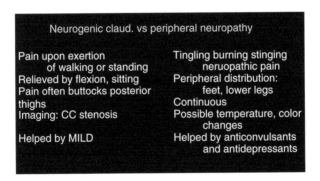

Fig. 3.21 The characteristics of neurogenic claudication vs. peripheral neuropathy

complaining more of radiculopathy than neurogenic claudication. The high incidence of LSS and the lack of an effective treatment without the disadvantages of a complex open spinal surgery has continued to generate interest in alternative therapies such as MILD.

3.9 MILD Literature Summary

In 2010, Chopko and Caraway reported the initial results of 78 patients treated for LSS with MILD as part of a non-randomized trial [12]. In 2013, Chopko reported the 2-year results from this trial [13]. At 6 weeks after treatment, the 75 patients available for follow-up reported significantly improvement in the mean visual ana-log pain scale (VAS) from 7.3 to 3.7 and in the mean Oswestry Disability Index (ODI) from 47.4 to 29.5. Lesser, but still significant, improvements were noted among the 45 patients available for 2-year follow-up, mean VAS 4.8 and mean ODI 39.8. The clinical improvement achieved was comparable to that reported from results of laminectomy in the SPORT trial [9]. No significant adverse events were reported. In contrast, the complications of laminectomy reported in the SPORT trial included a 9 % incidence of dural tear or spinal fluid leak and 2 % incidence of wound infection. The average length of stay for the laminectomy procedure was 3.5 days vs. zero for the outpatient MILD procedures.

In 2010, Lingreen and Grider reported their retrospective experience with 42 consecutive patients treated for LSS with the MILD technique [14]. Bilateral MILD procedures were performed at one (n = 14), two (n = 26), or three (n = 2) lumbar lev-els. The preoperative mean VAS was 9.6, which decreased significantly to 5.8 at 30 days. Only one patient reported the ability to ambulate for > 15 min prior to the onset of neurogenic claudication prior to surgery, while 25 (60 %) of patients could do so 30 days after surgery. No significant complications were reported.

In 2011 Schomer et al. reported a multicenter, retrospective review of acute safety and short-term efficacy from patients treated with the MILD procedure at multiple institutions [15]. Acute safety data was available for 253 patients; no sig-nificant complications were reported. Three month outcome data were available for 107 patients. The mean baseline VAS was 7.4, which decreased significantly to 3.9. The mean baseline ODI was 48.0, which decreased significantly to 30.9.

In 2012, Basu reported the results of a prospective, non-randomized trial of 27 patients treated for LSS with the MILD technique [16]. Mild procedures were per-formed at one (n = 10) or two levels (n = 17); all except one procedure were bilateral. At 6-month follow-up, the mean baseline VAS of 9.1 had decreased significantly to 3.9. The mean baseline ODI was 55.1, which decreased significantly to 31.1. No significant complications were reported.

In 2012, Wong reported the results of a prospective, non-randomized seventeen patient MILD case series [17]. He reported significant improvement in the mean VAS from 7.6 to 2.3 and in the mean ODI from 48.4 to 21.7 at 1 year. He reported no significant complications.

Deer et al. reported the results of a single center prospective, non-randomized trial of 46 patients treated with MILD in 2012 [18]. MILD procedures were per-formed at one (n = 24) or two levels (n = 22). Procedures were bilateral at 44 levels and unilateral at 24 levels. Patients were followed up to 1 year after treatment, with complete follow-up data available for 35 patients. For the 35 patients with complete follow-up, they reported significant improvement in the mean VAS from 6.9 to 4.0 and in the mean ODI from 49.4 to 32.0 at 1 year. No serious complications were reported.

In 2012, Brown reported the results of a double-blind, randomized trial of epi-dural steroid injection vs. MILD for LSS in a group of 38 patients [19]. Twenty one patients were initially treated with MILD and 17 with epidural injections. At 6 weeks post treatment, the mean VAS scores for the MILD group improved from 6.3 to 3.8, with 16 (76 %) patients improving by more than two points. The mean ODI improved from 38.8 to 27.4. At the same time point, the mean VAS scores for the epidural injection group remained essentially unchanged, with only 6 (35 %) improving by more than two points. The mean ODI improved slightly from 40.5 to 34.8. All of the epidural patients eventually crossed to the MILD group, many doing so before 12 weeks. The mean VAS in the crossover group improved from 7.4 to 4.5. No significant complications were reported.

Mekhail et al. reported the results of a single center prospective, non-randomized trial of 40 patients treated with MILD in 2012 [20]. Fifty-three MILD procedures were performed at one (n = 27) or two levels (n = 13). The procedures were bilateral at 37 levels and unilateral at 16 levels. Thirty-four patients completed follow-up through 1 year. Two of the six patients without complete follow-up underwent subsequent open surgical procedures. For the 34 patients with 1-year follow-up, the mean VAS improved significantly from 7.1 to 3.6. The Pain Disability Index improved significantly from 41.4 to 18.8. The Roland-Morris Disability Index also improved significantly from 14.3 to 6.6. No serious complications were reported.

The MiDAS III trial recently enrolled 138 patients in a prospective, non-randomized trial for treatment of LSS with the MILD technique. Results of this trial have not been reported to date. To date, there has not been a randomized trial directly comparing MILD to open surgical laminectomy.

In summary, all published reports of treatment of LSS with the MILD technique support an excellent safety profile. We found no published reports of dural tear, infection, death, or other serious complication associated with a MILD procedure, in contrast to the 9 % dural tear and 2 % infection rates reported from the SPORT trial [9]. The multiple published series also demonstrate short-term clinical outcomes comparable to those achieved with open laminectomy. In the SPORT LSS surgical cohort of 394 patients, the mean ODI improved significantly from 43.2 to 21.8. In this same group, the Low Back Pain Bothersomeness Index (LBPBI) also improved significantly from 4.1 to 2.1. The LBPBI is a six-point scale comparable to the VAS reported in most MILD series. Although some might consider laminectomy to be a definitive and durable treatment for LSS, the SPORT trial also reported that 13 % of patients underwent additional spine surgery within a 4-year period.

3.10   A Surgeon's Perspective

The MILD procedure is a radical departure from the conventional wisdom surrounding the surgical treatment of lumbar spinal stenosis. In essence, the MILD procedure is a remodeling, as well as a resection, of the hypertrophic ligamentum flavum. This remodeling and partial resection leads to a thinned ligament, which is partially if not completely disinserted from its attachments to the laminar edges. As a result, the ligament is untethered, allowing relaxation of the ligament in the dorsal direction, which contributes to the anatomic relief of stenosis.

Classically, a decompressive laminectomy can be described as a clear-cutting or "scorched earth" procedure, whereby every element dorsal and dorsolateral to the dura is resected in its entirety. The end result is a spinal canal where the glistening dorsal aspect of the theca is all that remains; lamina, spinous process, associated paraspinal muscles and ligaments, and even the medial component of the facet joints are all now absent. In a case of central spinal stenosis, the MILD procedure begs a different and tantalizing question, namely, what is the minimum amount of dorsal element tissue that needs to be resected in order to achieve a positive clinical result?

A percutaneous, minimally disruptive procedure such as MILD has myriad potential benefits:

1. High patient acceptance
2. Lack of paraspinal muscular disruption
3. Complete preservation of the facet joints
4. The option to perform the procedure under local anesthesia and minimal sedation
5. The lack of a need for thermal cautery, which diminishes wound healing complications such as seroma formation
6. Avoidance of blood transfusion
7. Minimal wound healing issues, as the working tract behaves exactly as a needle tract and tends to self-seal upon removal of the cannula
8. Avoidance of need for inpatient hospitalization

Due to the intrinsic minimally invasive nature of the procedure, MILD is well suited for treatment of patients who are otherwise deemed to be poor candidates for conventional open spinal surgery on account of medical comorbidities. Multiple MILD trials have demonstrated the safety of the procedure, a finding which has been replicated in a high-risk patient population [21, 22].

As with all surgical procedures, outcome success is dependent on appropriate patient selection. The MILD procedure has no role in the treatment of lateral recess or foraminal stenosis, discogenic compression, or patients in whom instrumentation, stabilization, and fusion is indicated. That said, the MILD procedure does indeed contribute a valid, alternative approach to the treatment of neurogenic claudication secondary to central canal stenosis due primarily to ligamentum flavum hypertrophy.

References

1. Deyo RA, Mirza SK, Martin BI. Back pain prevalence and visit rates. Spine. 2006;31:2724–7.
2. Deyo RA, Weinstein JN. Low back pain. N Engl J Med. 2001;344:363–70.
3. Kalichman L, Cole R, Kim DH, et al. Spinal stenosis prevalence and association with symptoms: the Framingham study. Spine J. 2009;9:545–50.
4. Kawaguchi Y, Kanamori M, Ishihara H, et al. Clinical and radiographic results of expansive lumbar laminoplasty in patients with spinal stenosis. J Bone Joint Surg Am. 2004; 86:1698–703.
5. Benz RJ, Ibrahim ZG, Afshar P, et al. Predicting complications in elderly patients undergoing lumbar decompression. Clin Orthop Relat Res. 2001;384:116–21.
6. Katz JN, Lipson SJ, Chang LC, et al. Seven to 10-year outcome of decompressive surgery for degenerative lumbar spinal stenosis. Spine. 1996;21:92–8.

7. Johnsson KE, Willner S, Johnsson K. Postoperative instability after decompression for lumbar spinal stenosis. Spine. 1986;11:107–10.
8. Sihvonen T, Herno A, Paljärvi L, et al. Local denervation atrophy of paraspinal muscles in postoperative failed back syndrome. Spine. 1993;18:575–81.
9. Weinstein JN, et al. Surgical versus nonoperative treatment for lumbar spinal stenosis. Four year results of the spine patient outcomes research trial. Spine. 2010;35:1329–38.
10. Burnett MR, et al. Cost-effectiveness of current treatment strategies for lumbar spinal stenosis: nonsurgical care, laminectomy, and X-STOP. J Neurosurg Spine. 2010;13(1):39–46.
11. Patil CG, et al. Interspinous device versus laminectomy for lumbar spinal stenosis: a comparative effectiveness study. Spine J. 2013;pii: S1529–9430(13)01501-5.
12. Chopko B, Caraway DL. MIDAS 1 (mild® decompression alternative to open surgery): a preliminary report of a prospective, multi-center clinical study. Pain Physician. 2010;13:369–78.
13. Chopko B. Long-term results of percutaneous lumbar decompression for LSS, two-year outcomes. Clin J Pain. 2013;29(11):939–43.
14. Lingreen R, Grider JS. Retrospective review of patient self-reported improvement and post-procedure findings for MILD (minimally invasive lumbar decompression). Pain Physician. 2010;13:555–60.
15. Schomer DF, Solsberg D, Wong W, Chopko BW. MILD lumbar decompression for the treatment of spinal stenosis. Neuroradiol J. 2011;24:620–6.
16. Basu S. MILD procedure: single-site prospective IRB study. Clin J Pain. 2011;28(3):254–8.
17. Wong W. Mild interlaminar decompression for the treatment of lumbar spinal stenosis, procedure description and case series with 1-year follow-up. Clin J Pain. 2012;28(6):534–8.
18. Deer TR, Kim CK, Bowman II RG, et al. Study of percutaneous lumbar decompression and treatment algorithm for patients suffering from neurogenic claudication. Pain Physician. 2012;15:451–60.
19. Brown LL. A double-blind, randomized, prospective study of epidural steroid injection vs. the mild® procedure in patients with symptomatic lumbar spinal stenosis. Pain Pract. 2012;12(5):333–41.
20. Mekhail N, Costandi S, Abraham B, Samuel SW. Functional and patient-reported outcomes in symptomatic lumbar spinal stenosis following percutaneous decompression. Pain Pract. 2012;12(6):417–25.
21. Chopko BW. A novel method for treatment of lumbar spinal stenosis in high-risk surgical candidates: pilot study experience with percutaneous remodeling of ligamentum flavum and lamina. J Neurosurg Spine. 2011;14:46–50.
22. Levy RM, Deer TR. Systematic safety review and meta-analysis of procedural experience using percutaneous access to treat symptomatic lumbar spinal stenosis. Pain Med. 2012;13:154–1561.

Pedicle-Lengthening Osteotomy for the Treatment of Lumbar Spinal Stenosis

4

D. Greg Anderson

4.1 Introduction

Lumbar spinal stenosis (LSS) remains the most common indication for spinal surgery in the older adult population [1]. Degenerative changes in the vertebral column including the intervertebral disc, facet joints, and ligamentum flavum can lead to a reduction in the diameter of the spinal canal, causing compression of the neural elements and producing symptoms of pain or neurologic dysfunction [2, 3]. Although nonsurgical treatments are generally attempted for this patient population, many patients with severe symptoms may not achieve sufficient relief and therefore require surgical intervention [4]. The most common surgical approach for LSS has been the open lumbar laminectomy [5]. Patients with associated degenerative spondylolisthesis are often treated with arthrodesis in addition to a laminectomy decompression [6].

Open lumbar laminectomy is capable of reducing the symptoms of LSS but is moderately invasive and may not be tolerated by some older patients with significant medical comorbidities [5]. The initial favorable results of open lumbar laminectomy have been shown to deteriorate over time and, in some cases, require revision surgery [7]. Minimally invasive surgical approaches for LSS have been utilized; however these techniques have not gained wide acceptance due to concerns over the steep learning curve and/or the potential for an inadequate decompression or a technical complication [8–12]. Interspinous spacers have also been used in the subset of LSS patients who achieve good symptom relief while sitting [13]. Unfortunately, concerns over the durability of this approach have limited the popularity of interspinous spacers [14–16].

D.G. Anderson, M.D.
Departments of Orthopaedic and Neurological Surgery, Thomas Jefferson University and Rothman Institute, 925 Chestnut St., 5th Floor, Philadelphia, PA 19107, USA
e-mail: greg.anderson@rothmaninstitute.com

© Springer International Publishing Switzerland 2016
L. Manfrè (ed.), *Spinal Canal Stenosis*, New Procedures in Spinal Interventional Neuroradiology, DOI 10.1007/978-3-319-26270-3_4

The pedicle-lengthening osteotomy procedure is a relatively new percutaneous surgical approach for LSS. To perform this procedure, the surgeon utilizes fluoroscopic guidance to cannulate the pedicles of the affected level(s). An internal passage is reamed through each pedicle into the vertebral body, leaving the cortical shell of the pedicle intact. A specialized handsaw is used to cut through the cortical shell of the pedicle (from inside the pedicle passage) at the junction of the pedicle and vertebral body. A specialized bone screw is threaded into the pedicle passage. The bone screw creates a gap (produces 4 mm of distraction) at the pedicle osteotomy site. The elongated pedicle heals, following the procedure, producing a permanent expansion of the spinal canal and neural foramina [17].

4.2   Surgical Technique

Pedicle-lengthening osteotomies are performed at lumbar levels requiring neural decompression. The selection of the surgical levels begins with a thorough history and physical examination of the patient. Advanced imaging studies (MRI or CT myelography) are always reviewed as part of the evaluation, and the location of nerve compression is correlated to the patient's clinical symptoms to determine the symptomatic levels of lumbar stenosis. All areas of clinically symptomatic nerve root compression should be included in the surgical plan.

To decompress a particular lumbar level, the pedicles above and below the symptomatic disc level are lengthened. For instance if the patient's symptoms are due to stenosis of the L4/L5 level, the surgeon should lengthen the L4 and L5 pedicles to correct the pathologic condition. The pedicle-lengthening osteotomy procedures may be performed under general anesthesia or local anesthesia and intravenous sedation. In either case, the patient is positioned prone on a radiolucent operating table with good access for fluoroscopic imaging. Surgeons may use either uniplanar or biplanar fluoroscopy during the pedicle-lengthening procedure, and some surgeons have utilized computer-assisted image guidance to perform the procedure.

After a sterile preparation and draping of the patient, fluoroscopic imaging is utilized to identify the pedicles to be lengthened. Using the *en face* fluoroscopic view, the site of the skin incision is demarcated directly in line with the central axis of the pedicle (Fig. 4.1). A 10 mm skin incision is made in line with the central axis of each pedicle. Next, a trochar-tipped reamer is utilized to cannulate the pedicle. It is important that the tip of the reamer be positioned within 2 mm of the center of the pedicle as seen on the *en face* view to ensure a well-centered passage through the pedicle is achieved. The reamer is passed down the center of the pedicle until the radiographic marker is positioned at the junction of the pedicle and vertebral body (Fig. 4.2). The reamer is then removed and the pedicle saw is placed into the pedicle passage (Fig. 4.3).

The pedicle saw is a hand-powered instrument that has a semiflexible saw blade that extends from the side of the saw shaft to cut the pedicle bone from inside the pedicle passage. The site of the pedicle osteotomy is located at the junction of the pedicle and vertebral body. With the pedicle saw positioned correctly, the surgeon

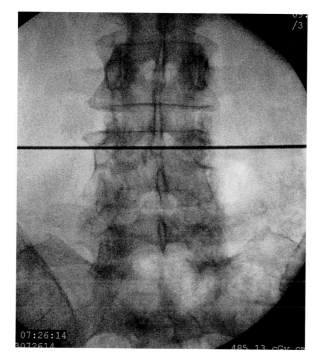

Fig. 4.1   An *en face* fluoroscopic view of the left L4 pedicle is shown with a Kirschner wire above the skin to demarcate the location of the pedicle for the planning of the skin incision

advances the blade in 1/8th mm increments by turning a knob on the upper portion of the saw. The saw is rotated within the pedicle passage to cut the pedicle bone at the site of the pedicle osteotomy. The initial 1–2 mm of the bone cut is performed with circumferential rotation of the pedicle saw. The remainder of the pedicle wall is cut with zonal cutting (Fig. 4.4). During zonal cutting, the pedicle is divided into four or more zones that are cut independently. This produces more accurate cutting of the uneven shape of the pedicle walls and reduces the risk of "past pointing" of the blade during the cutting procedure. As the pedicle saw blade is extended in 1/8th mm increments during cutting, the blade should be swept across the internal bony walls of the pedicle until the outer cortex of the pedicle wall has been breached. The blade is then retracted and the saw is adjusted to cut the next pedicle zone. Throughout the cutting procedure, the saw provides excellent tactile feedback allowing the surgeon to "feel" the sensation of the saw blade scraping away thin layers of bone. With experience, the surgeon will be able to detect the tactile sensation of the saw blade breaching the wall of the pedicle in a reliable fashion. Throughout the pedicle cutting process, periodic fluoroscopy images in the *en face* and lateral projections are obtained to check the position of the saw blade relative to the outer cortex of the pedicle (Fig. 4.5).

During pedicle cutting, the primary "at risk" structure is the traversing nerve root that courses along the medical and interior walls of the pedicle. The surgeon must use

Fig. 4.2 A trochar-tipped
bone reamer is passed
through the central region
of the pedicle until the
radiographic marker (notch
at the waist of the reamer)
reaches the base of the
pedicle

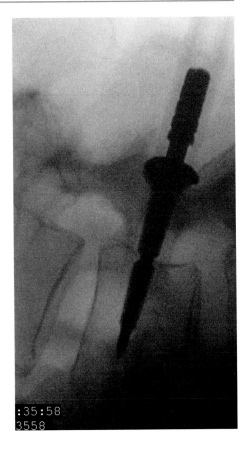

particular care in these regions to ensure that the blade of the saw does not project
significantly beyond the walls of the pedicle. The geometry of the saw blade is
designed to reduce the potential for nerve injury in the event of contact between the
blade tip and nerve root. In addition, the surgeon may use stimulated EMG monitoring to assist in detecting any contact between the blade and nerve root.

After cutting the pedicles, an expandable bone screw is threaded into the pedicles
and positioned utilizing the radiographic marker at the site of the pedicle cut (Fig. 4.6).
A threaded mechanism is then used to lengthen the screw implant causing expansion
of the gap at the base of the pedicle to 4 mm (Fig. 4.7). The bone screw locks in the
expanded position to prevent loss of pedicle lengthening and maintain the lengthened
position of the pedicle until bone healing across the osteotomy transpires (Fig. 4.8).

After completing the procedure, final fluoroscopic imaging is utilized to confirm
position of the pedicle-lengthening devices. The surgical incisions are closed and
local anesthetic is injected subcutaneously at the surgical sites for postoperative
pain management. Patients are mobilized rapidly after recovery from anesthesia and
encouraged to resume normal daily activities except for bending or twisting of the
lumbar area for the first 6 weeks to allow bone healing at the osteotomy sites.

Fig. 4.3 A specialized hand-powered bone saw is placed into the pedicle passage and used to cut the pedicle at the junction of the pedicle and vertebral body

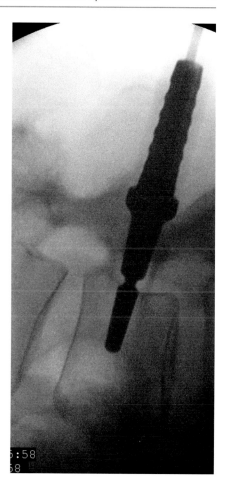

4.3   Discussion

Lumbar spinal stenosis is an increasingly common condition, due to aging of the population [2]. The rate of surgery for LSS varies widely in different regions of the world. Jansson and colleagues reported a rate of surgery for lumbar stenosis of 13.2 per 100,000 Swedish citizens in 1999 and noted a threefold increase between 1987 and 1999 [18]. In contrast, the rate of lumbar decompression surgery declined slightly between 2002 and 2007 for the US Medicare population [19].

The SPORT study provided multicentered, prospective outcome data on patients with LSS with and without a concomitant low-grade degenerative spondylolisthesis. In the SPORT study, patients with LSS were treated with a decompressive lumbar laminectomy, and lumbar fusion was added for the subset of patients with degenerative spondylolisthesis. Surgical care was also compared to a course of usual nonoperative care [20]. In the cohort without spondylolisthesis,

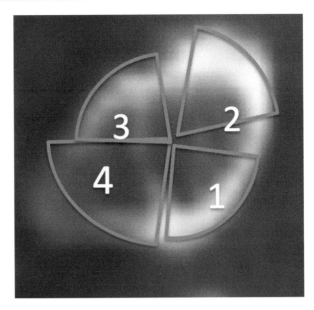

Fig. 4.4 Coronal reconstruction of a pedicle demonstrates an asymmetric pedicle shape. The pedicle is cut in zones (orange pie-shaped regions) to reduce "past pointing" of the bone saw blade

the 24-month as-treated analysis demonstrated a mean improvement of 16.1 (±1.9) points compared to the mean baseline Oswestry Disability Index (ODI) scores. This was statistically superior to the improvement of 12.7 (±1.8) points on

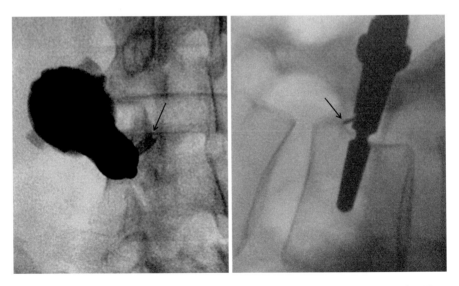

Fig. 4.5 *En face* and lateral fluoroscopic images of the pedicle saw during pedicle cutting. Note the location of the saw blade (*arrows*) is easily seen relative to the margins of the pedicle wall

Fig. 4.6 Bone screw in place in the pedicle before expansion of the bone screw. Notice the slight gap where the pedicle cut has been performed

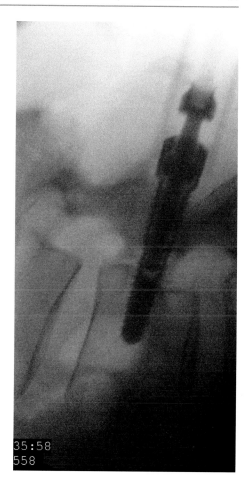

the ODI scale for the nonoperative cohort. The SPORT study reported blood transfusions in 15 % and dural tears in 9 % of patients treated by lumbar laminectomy. Patients undergoing a concomitant lumbar fusion had a higher rate of complications including blood transfusion (35 % intraoperative and 16 % postoperative), dural tears (12 %), wound infection (5 %), and additional surgery within 12 months (8 %) [20].

Complication rates and clinical outcome following lumbar laminectomy surgery have been reported by other authors. Deyo et al. studied Medicare claims and reported life-threatening complications in 2.3–5.6 % of patients undergoing surgery for LSS depending on the invasiveness of the surgical approach. An additional 7.8–13 % of the LSS cases required hospital readmission within the first 30 days of surgery [19]. Reoperation rates following laminectomy for LSS were reported to be 23 % within 8–10 years in the prospective, observational Maine cohort study [21]. In a 7–10 year follow-up study, Katz et al. reported a 33 % rate of severe back pain following open lumbar decompression [7].

Fig. 4.7 The bone screw
after expansion showing
lengthening of the pedicle
and enlargement of the
spinal canal

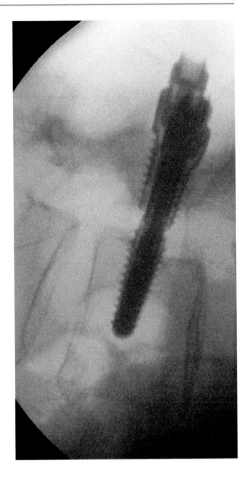

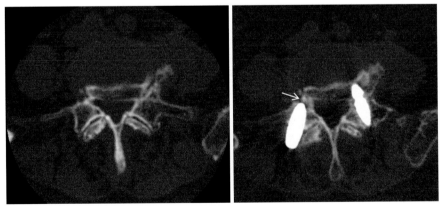

Fig. 4.8 Computed tomography scan of the L5 level before and after pedicle lengthening. Notice
the increase space in the lateral recess of the spinal canal. Also notice, the healing of the pedicle
osteotomy (*arrow*)

Minimally invasive techniques for lumbar decompression have become increasingly popular in recent years. These procedures often employ a tubular retractor system which limits the soft tissue disruption of the surgical approach [8]. Rahman et al. reported less blood loss, reduced operating times, shorter hospital stays, and a lower rate of complications in a cohort of patients following minimally invasive decompression when compared to open decompression [22]. Rigorous prospective studies comparing the outcome of open laminectomy to minimally invasive decompression are currently lacking [23, 24]. Only two small studies could be found which prospectively compare minimally invasive surgical decompression to open decompression [25, 26]. In a retrospective data mining study, Fu et al. reported lower rates of death and neurological complications among enrollees of the Scoliosis Research Society database treated with a minimally invasive approach as compared to open surgery [27]. Despite these encouraging reports, concerns persist among many surgeons regarding the steep learning curve and risk of technical complication due to inadequate visualization with minimally invasive techniques. [26] These concerns have currently limited the adoption of minimally invasive decompression techniques.

Interspinous spacers have been studied for selected cases of LSS. In the United States, the X-Stop device (Medtronic Spine, Sunnyvale, California) was approved by the Food and Drug Administration in 2005 for the treatment of LSS and has achieved mixed results. Although one large trial showed the X-Stop to be superior to nonoperative care [28], others have reported problems with the device. For instance, Brussee et al. found that only 31 % of their patient cohort achieved a good result following X-Stop implantation [14]. Tuschel et al. reported a 30 % revision rate, mostly in the first year after implantation, due to inadequate relief from the symptoms of stenosis [29]. Kim et al. found spinous process fractures in 29 % of the cases in their series [15]. Bowers et al. reported complications in 38 % of patients and performed revision surgery in 85 % of the patients in their series [16]. Because of these concerns, intraspinous spacers have not replaced open lumbar decompression as the predominant method of treatment for LSS at the current time.

The pedicle-lengthening osteotomy procedure provides a novel surgical strategy for enlarging the spinal canal and neural foramen using a percutaneous approach. The theoretical advantages of this procedure include the lack of removal of normal anatomic structures and the reduced risk of major bleeding, infection, and medical complications compared to traditional open lumbar decompression. A compelling aspect of pedicle lengthening is the lack of removal of normal anatomic structures which should limit the risks of postoperative instability. Mlyavykh et al. reported the results of a pilot study for pedicle lengthening which demonstrated favorable clinical results and a low perioperative complication rate [30]. Further study of this technique and a more direct comparison to alternative treatment strategies for lumbar spinal stenosis will be needed in the future to define the ultimate role of this procedure for the treatment of lumbar spinal stenosis.

References

1. Atlas SJ, Keller RB, Robson D, et al. Surgical and nonsurgical management of lumbar spinal stenosis: four-year outcomes from the maine lumbar spine study. Spine. 2000;25:556–62.
2. Siebert E, Pruss H, Klingebiel R, et al. Lumber spinal stenosis: syndrome, diagnostics and treatment. Nat Rev Neurol. 2009;5:392–403.
3. Weinstein JN, Tosteson TD, Lurie JD, et al. Surgical versus nonsurgical therapy for lumbar spinal stenosis. N Engl J Med. 2008;358:794–810.
4. Yuan PS, Albert TJ. Nonsurgical and surgical management of lumbar spinal stenosis. J Bone Joint Surg Am. 2004;86:2320–30.
5. Fredman B, Arinzon Z, Zohar E, et al. Observations on the safety and efficacy of surgical decompression for lumbar spinal stenosis in geriatric patients. Eur Spine J: Off Publ Eur Spine Soc, Eur Spinal Deformity Soc, Eur Sect Cervical Spine Res Soc. 2002;11(6):571–4.
6. Herkowitz HN, Kurz LT. Degenerative lumbar spondylolisthesis with spinal stenosis: a prospective study comparing decompression with decompression and intertransverse process arthrodesis. J Bone Joint Surg Am. 1991;73:802–8.
7. Katz JN, Lipson SJ, Chang LC, et al. Seven to 10-year outcome of decompressive surgery for degenerative lumbar spinal stenosis. Spine. 1996;21(1):92–8.
8. Asgarzadie F, Khoo LT. Minimally invasive operative management for lumbar spinal stenosis: overview of early and long-term outcomes. Orthop Clin North Am. 2007;38(3):387–99.
9. Hamasaki T, Tanaka N, Kim J, et al. Biomechanical assessment of minimally invasive decompression for lumbar spinal canal stenosis: a cadaver study. J Spinal Disord Tech. 2009;22(7): 486–91.
10. Podichetty VK, Spears J, Isaacs RE, et al. Complications associated with minimally invasive decompression for lumbar spinal stenosis. J Spinal Disord Tech. 2006;19(3):161–6.
11. Rahimi-Movaghar V, Rasouli MR, Vaccaro AR. Patient outcomes vs a minimally invasive approach in lumbar spinal stenosis: which is more important? Neurosurgery. 2010;67(4):E1180.
12. Yoshimoto M, Takebayashi T, Kawaguchi S, et al. Minimally invasive technique for decompression of lumbar foraminal stenosis using a spinal microendoscope: technical note. Minim Invasive Neurosurg: MIN. 2011;54(3):142–6.
13. Kondrashov DG, Hannibal M, Hsu KY, Zucherman JF. Interspinous process decompression with the X-STOP device for lumbar spinal stenosis: a 4-year follow-up study. J Spinal Disord Tech. 2006;19(5):323–7.
14. Brussee P, Hauth J, Donk RD, et al. Self-rated evaluation of outcome of the implantation of interspinous process distraction (X-Stop) for neurogenic claudication. Eur Spine J: Off Publ Eur Spine Soc, Eur Spinal Deformity Soc, Eur Sect Cervical Spine Res Soc. 2008; 17(2):200–3.
15. Kim DH, Tantorski M, Shaw J, et al. Occult spinous process fractures associated with interspinous process spacers. Spine. 2011;36(16):E1080–5.
16. Bowers C, Amini A, Dailey AT, et al. Dynamic interspinous process stabilization: review of complications associated with the X-Stop device. Neurosurg Focus. 2010;28(6):E8.
17. Kiapour A, Anderson DG, Spenciner DB, et al. Kinematic effects of a pedicle-lengthening osteotomy for the treatment of lumbar spinal stenosis. J Neurosurg Spine. 2012;17(4): 314–20.
18. Jansson KA, Blomqvist P, Granath F, Nemeth G. Spinal stenosis surgery in Sweden 1987–1999. Eur Spine J: Off Publ Eur Spine Soc, Eur Spinal Deformity Soc, Eur Sect Cervical Spine Res Soc. 2003;12(5):535–41.
19. Deyo RA, Mirza SK, Martin BI, Kreuter W, Goodman DC, Jarvik JG. Trends, major medical complications, and charges associated with surgery for lumbar spinal stenosis in older adults. JAMA. 2010;303(13):1259–65.
20. Weinstein JN, Tosteson TD, Lurie JD, et al. Surgical versus nonoperative treatment for lumbar spinal stenosis four-year results of the spine patient outcomes research trial. Spine. 2010;35(14):1329–38.

21. Atlas SJ, Keller RB, Wu YA, et al. Long-term outcomes of surgical and nonsurgical management of lumbar spinal stenosis: 8 to 10 year results from the maine lumbar spine study. Spine. 2005;30(8):936–43.
22. Rahman M, Summers LE, Richter B, et al. Comparison of techniques for lumbar laminectomy: the minimally invasive versus the "classic" open approach. Minim Invasive Neurosurg. 2008; 51:100–5.
23. Fu KM, Smith JS, Polly Jr DW, et al. Morbidity and mortality in the surgical treatment of 10,329 adults with degenerative lumbar stenosis. J Neurosurg Spine. 2010;12(5):443–6.
24. Mannion RJ, Guilfoyle MR, Efendy J, et al. Minimally invasive lumbar decompression: long-term outcome, morbidity, and the learning curve from the first 50 cases. J Spinal Disord Tech. 2012;25(1):47–51.
25. Rosen DS, O'Toole JE, Eichholz KM, et al. Minimally invasive lumbar spinal decompression in the elderly: outcomes of 50 patients aged 75 years and older. Neurosurgery. 2007; 60(3):503–9.
26. Lauryssen C. Technical advances in minimally invasive surgery: direct decompression for lumbar spinal stenosis. Spine. 2010;35(26):S287–93.
27. Stucki G, Daltroy L, Liang MH, et al. Measurement properties of a self-administered outcome measure in lumbar spinal stenosis. Spine. 1996;21(7):796–803.
28. Zucherman JF, Hsu KY, Hartjen CA, et al. A prospective randomized multi-center study for the treatment of lumbar spinal stenosis with the X STOP interspinous implant: 1-year results. Eur Spine J. 2004;13(1):22–31.
29. Tuschel A, Chavanne A, Eder C, Meissl M, Becker P, Ogon M. Implant survival analysis and failure modes of the X-Stop interspinous distraction device. Spine (Phila Pa 1976). 2013;1;38(21):1826–31.
30. Mlyavykh S, Ludwig SC, Mobasser JP, Kepler CK, Anderson DG. Twelve-month results of a clinical pilot study utilizing pedicle-lengthening osteotomy for the treatment of lumbar spinal stenosis. J Neurosurg Spine. 2013;18(4):347–55.

Technical Considerations in Percutaneous Placement of Spinal Cord Stimulation Devices

Edwin Gulko, Todd Miller, and Allan Brook

5.1 Introduction

The last several decades have witnessed exponential advances in the technology and use of spinal cord neuromodulation for the treatment of chronic refractory pain syndromes in patients whom medical and surgical management have been exhausted. This chapter focuses on the technical aspects of percutaneous placement of SCN devices, emphasizing patient selection, technique, and complications.

The precise mechanism of spinal cord modulation for neuropathic pain is partially understood. The original "control gate theory" postulated that continual activation of afferent fibers within the dorsal columns of the spinal cord inhibited transmission of nociceptive stimulation [1]. The basis of SCN was rooted in this theory and currently serves as the framework for explaining the benefits of SCN. However, it is believed that a more complex interweave between neuronal activity at the dorsal horn, involvement of supraspinal circuits, and modulation of neurotransmitters within the dorsal horn are also involved [1, 2]. The benefits of SCN for refractory angina, other ischemic diseases, and CRPS (Complex Regional Pain Syndrome) are felt to be secondary to a different set of mechanisms [1]. In all cases, the goal is to replace the pain sensation with a paresthesia or tingling sensation (and more recently with high-frequency modulation without the paresthesias). The goal is decreased pain with less medication resulting in greater mobility and quality of life.

Abundant data is available supporting the role for spinal cord neuromodulation (SCN). In a prospective randomized control study performed by North et al. among patients with prior lumbosacral surgeries (failed back surgery syndrome)

E. Gulko, M.D. • T. Miller, M.D. (✉) • A. Brook, M.D.
Department of Radiology, Diagnostic and Interventional Neuroradiology, Albert Einstein College of Medicine, Montefiore Medical Center, Bronx, NY, USA
e-mail: edwin.gulko@gmail.com; tmiller@montefiore.org; abrook2214@aol.com

© Springer International Publishing Switzerland 2016
L. Manfrè (ed.), *Spinal Canal Stenosis*, New Procedures in Spinal Interventional Neuroradiology, DOI 10.1007/978-3-319-26270-3_5

who met clinical and imaging criteria for additional surgical intervention, spinal cord stimulation was found to be more effective than reoperation during the study time period [3].

The PROCESS study was a randomized multicenter controlled study that aimed to evaluate the efficacy of spinal cord stimulation added to medical management, compared to medical management alone in patients with failed back surgery syndrome and radicular leg pain, with the primary outcome being pain relief [4]. Initial follow-up at 6 months demonstrated better primary outcome measures as well as other quality of life and functional capacity measures [5]. Patients initially randomized to the spinal cord stimulation arm were followed out to 24 months, excluding any patients that crossed over into spinal cord stimulation group. Unfortunately the number of remaining patients initially randomized to the conservative medical management group was deemed too small for comparative analyses. Regardless, Kumar et al. demonstrated that pain relief was sustained in patients with spinal cord stimulation [6].

5.2   Patient Selection

As with any procedure, patient selection and an understanding of contraindications for SCN are crucial components of obtaining favorable outcomes. Appropriate patient selection begins by identifying a clear etiology for the patient's source of pain; SCN is typically sought after conservative pain management measures have failed [7].

The more common indications include failed back surgery syndrome, complex regional pain syndrome (including causalgia and reflex sympathetic dystrophy), refractory angina pectoris, peripheral vascular disease, and post-amputation pain syndromes [7, 8].

Some contraindications include psychiatric instability, pain as a result of an accident in litigation, alcohol or drug addiction, pregnancy, coagulopathy, and inability to maintain/care for the device secondary to dementia or a psychiatric condition [7–9]. The Neuromodulation Appropriateness Consensus Committee lists indications, cautions, and inappropriate practices [9].

5.3   Technique

5.3.1   Trial

A trial period with temporary leads is performed to determine if the procedure provides adequate relief before permanent implantation. This allows for an enhanced level of appropriate patient selection. Patient education and cooperation are crucial, as both self-monitoring of symptoms and effective communication with the physician help judge the degree of trial success. The trial procedure consists of temporary percutaneous lead placement and connection to the pulse generator, which is maintained in a wearable elastic pouch. This allows the patient to judge success in their own environment doing their daily activities.

The patient is placed in the prone position on the fluoroscopy table and skin prepped in sterile fashion. Per recommendations from the Neuromodulation Appropriateness Consensus Committee of the International Neuromodulation Society, real-time interaction between the patient and physician is the ideal circumstance under which to implant the electrodes [9]. Patient sedation must be titrated to provide comfort, while the patient maintains the ability to effectively describe the location and intensity of induced paresthesias. This promotes ideal lead localization. If general anesthesia is required, areas of lead coverage may be evaluated with somatosensory evoked potential monitoring [10].

Under flouroscopic guidance, an introducer needle is placed into the epidural space from a paramedian approach. A lead is introduced into the dorsal epidural space and guided to the appropriate level corresponding to the dermatomal distribution of pain. Depending on the practitioner's preference, one or two leads may be inserted. Electrode position at T1–T4 is adequate for upper extremity pain, with advancement of the lead as needed for appropriate coverage [8, 9]. Electrode position from T6 to T10 is usually adequate for back and lower limb pain [8], with the electrodes advanced in real time to target these regions [9].

At this point, the lead(s) can be attached to the external stimulator for testing. Modern electrodes have several channels, which allow for "tuning" of the stimulation field. This tuning allows the stimulation field to be tailored to the patient's needs without moving the electrode. Varying amplitudes are applied to discern when the patient first feels paresthesias (perception threshold) and when the magnitude of stimulation is intolerable (discomfort threshold). The difference between the two is the usage range [2]. The location of the lead(s) may need to be adjusted to insure appropriate dermatome coverage and limit motor stimulation which is typically felt as abdominal wall or chest muscle contractions depending on the area being treated. After the appropriate settings and positioning are obtained, the lead is sutured to the skin and covered with antibiotic ointment and sterile dressing. Leads are secured to the skin with interrupted sutures to prevent their dislodgment during the trial period. Sterile dressings are used to cover the entire apparatus to limit the opportunity for infection and further minimize movement, which may dislodge the leads. Antibiotics are administered pre- and post-procedure to cover the patient for the duration of the trial period.

A trial period lasting approximately 5 days is sufficient to determine if the treatment will provide adequate pain relief and functional improvement. During the trial, the patients perform daily activities and monitor the degree of symptomatic relief. The patient is provided with a diary where they record activity, pain, and various life quality measures.

After the trial, the patient returns to the office for removal of the electrode. The sutures are cut, and a gentle tug is sufficient to remove the electrode. A small gauze dressing is applied. Careful inspection is necessary to ensure that the entire electrode has been removed and that there is no sign of infection. Both of these facts are documented in the patient's record.

At this point, the patient and provider discuss the results. The patient is sent home for another week and is instructed to continue recording in the diary. The patient returns after the final week so a discussion and review of the diary can help guide the decision to proceed to permanent implant. An alternative approach is to conduct a trial period in the OR suite with a permanent electrode, with permanent placement if the desired affect is achieved [7]. Generally, a successful trial results in pain reduction by greater than 50 % [7, 8].

5.3.2 Permanent Placement: Percutaneous Leads

In most cases the process can be similar to the trial insertion. Cylinder-shaped permanent electrodes are placed percutaneously, with conscious sedation. This allows for intraoperative confirmation of proper position as with the trial placement. Paddle-type electrodes are placed surgically. These have a lower risk of migration, but require laminotomy for placement. Use of paddle type may be necessary if the epidural space has been compromised or the patient had prior laminectomy/posterior fusion [8, 9]. This should be evident after a percutaneous trial placement has been unsuccessful.

Prior (and for 7–10 days post) to the procedure, the patient is given antibiotics for coverage of skin flora. After proper lead placement, moderate sedation is recommended allowing for patient comfort during tunneling and generator placement.

Two needles are inserted into the epidural space through a paramedian approach depending on the targeted dermatome. They may be placed at different levels on the same side or on the same level on different sides of the midline. The former allows for only one incision during anchoring of the leads [8]. The electrodes are inserted and guided into the epidural space as with the trial. Electrode advancement should always be done under fluoroscopic guidance to ensure that leads do not course laterally or anteriorly. Two parallel electrodes provide more neural contacts at the midline [11]. Additionally the greater coverage along the neuroaxis allows for a greater range of programmable adjustments and tuning, as opposed to manual adjustment of electrode placement.

After proper lead positioning, test stimulation ensures that the patient experiences paresthesias in the corresponding regions of pain. Images should be obtained to document lead location. After the leads are manipulated into the desired locations, the skin area around the needle is anesthetized. An incision is made caudally or transversely if two needle insertions were created on either side of the midline. Gentle dissection is performed to expose the supraspinous ligament or paravertebral fascia. The needle and stylet are removed, and the electrodes are connected to anchors, which are fixed to supraspinous ligament with suture [8].

Additional local anesthetic is given from the midline out laterally, along a projected tunneling path. The lead tunneler is advanced subcutaneously in the lateral direction to the site where the pulse generator will be placed. The tunneler allows for passage of a straw device from the midline to the lateral exit site, where leads are then subsequently attached to the straw device and pulled laterally through the tunneled path out to the exit site. The skin incision is irrigated and closed with absorbable sutures for the subcutaneous tissues, and nylon sutures, liquid adhesive, and staples are used to close the skin [8].

Finally, a pocket is created for placement of the pulse generator. A 4 cm incision is made for the subcutaneous pocket superficial to the muscle layers. It is advisable to make the pocket less than 2 cm from the skin surface, to allow adequate communication with the electromagnetic programming device. After creation of the pocket, the leads are connected to the generator. The connection and functionality are tested, and the pulse generator is placed into the subcutaneous pocket. The pocket is irrigated and closed in standard surgical fashion with absorbable sutures for the subcutaneous tissues and nylon sutures, liquid adhesive, and staples for the skin [8].

5.4   Complications

A priori knowledge of potential technical challenges and complications prepares the physician during and after the procedure to negotiate and solve challenges that may arise. Placement of spinal cord stimulation devices for patients with failed back syndrome or complex regional pain syndrome is relatively safe with a low incidence of life-threatening complications. In over 130 percutaneous trials and placements in our lab, we have seen one CSF leak that occurred during a trial in a patient with failed back syndrome.

An exhaustive list of potential complications has been characterized and described by the Neuromodulation Appropriateness Consensus Committee and is categorized as: patient-related, device-related, technique-related, or biologic complications [10]. Common device-related complications include lead migration, fracture, and hardware malfunction [12]. Patient-related complications include infection, hematoma, CSF leaks, seromas, or pain [7, 8, 12].

Recognition of typical stimulation patterns is required to understand where an electrode may be positioned. Stimulation should be confined entirely to the dorsal columns, with paresthesias occurring ipsilateral and caudal to the electrode [13]. Stimulation patterns that result in abdominal tightness or chest wall sensations may indicate that a lead is positioned in the anterior epidural space. Intradural placement or placement adjacent to an exiting nerve root produces sensations that occur at extremely low amplitudes or within a narrow range [8].

Changes in regional anatomy of the axial spine pose varying challenges during electrode placement. Levy's manuscript, *Anatomic Considerations for Spinal Cord Stimulation*, eloquently details technical challenges that arise merely from anatomical variations that occur along the axial spine [13]. For instance, the cervical spinal cord is relatively thicker from C3 thru C7, the same levels that experience the greatest degree of degenerative changes. Consequently the possibility of spinal cord injury during epidural placement is the greatest at these levels, secondary to the smaller volume of the dorsal epidural space [13]. Additionally given the degree of motility to the cervical spine, changes in stimulation sensations are more likely secondary to lead displacement during cervical spinal motion [13].

Challenges posed in thoracic spine anatomy occur secondary to the varying positions of the spinal cord within the spinal canal. Secondary to the kyphotic curvature of the thoracic spine, the spinal cord lies in different ventral-dorsal positions depending on the thoracic level. Consequently the CSF thickness between spinal cord and epidural space also varies [13]. For low back pain, SCN lead placement typical is aimed at T8–T9 where the CSF space is relatively thick. As current from the electrodes travels along paths of least resistance, epidural stimulation at this level may activate fibers of the dorsal column but also of dorsal root fibers. Consequently patients may experience uncomfortable thoracic radicular sensations. Ventral and dorsal CSF thickness can change with varying patient positioning [14]. Consequently in patients with SCN devices, patient position (i.e., sitting/standing or lying) can affect stimulation sensations and efficacy [13].

The use of spinal cord stimulating devices has grown dramatically as the technology has improved in recent years. When patients are properly selected, the success rate is high, and complication rates are low. Percutaneous techniques are ideally suited to allow minimal sedation, which encourages patient report of sensations to guide optimal lead placement.

References

1. Linderoth B, Foreman RD. Physiology of spinal cord stimulation: review and update. Neuromodulation: J Int Neuromodulation Soc. 1999;2(3):150–64.
2. Oakley JC, Prager JP. Spinal cord stimulation: mechanisms of action. Spine. 2002; 27(22):2574–83.
3. North RB, Kidd DH, Farrokhi F, Piantadosi SA. Spinal cord stimulation versus repeated lumbosacral spine surgery for chronic pain: a randomized, controlled trial. Neurosurgery. 2005;56(1):98–106; discussion −7.
4. Kumar K, North R, Taylor R, Sculpher M, Van den Abeele C, Gehring M, et al. Spinal cord stimulation vs. conventional medical management: a prospective, randomized, controlled, multicenter study of patients with failed back surgery syndrome (PROCESS Study). Neuromodulation: J Int Neuromodulation Soc. 2005;8(4):213–8.
5. Kumar K, Taylor RS, Jacques L, Eldabe S, Meglio M, Molet J, et al. Spinal cord stimulation versus conventional medical management for neuropathic pain: a multicentre randomised controlled trial in patients with failed back surgery syndrome. Pain. 2007;132(1–2):179–88.
6. Kumar K, Taylor RS, Jacques L, Eldabe S, Meglio M, Molet J, et al. The effects of spinal cord stimulation in neuropathic pain are sustained: a 24-month follow-up of the prospective randomized controlled multicenter trial of the effectiveness of spinal cord stimulation. Neurosurgery. 2008;63(4):762–70; discussion 70.
7. Day M. Neuromodulation: spinal cord and peripheral nerve stimulation. Curr Rev Pain. 2000;4(5):374–82.
8. Brook AL, Georgy BA, Olan WJ. Spinal cord stimulation: a basic approach. Tech Vasc Interv Radiol. 2009;12(1):64–70.
9. Deer TR, Mekhail N, Provenzano D, Pope J, Krames E, Leong M, et al. The appropriate use of neurostimulation of the spinal cord and peripheral nervous system for the treatment of chronic pain and ischemic diseases: the neuromodulation appropriateness consensus committee. Neuromodulation : J Int Neuromodulation Soc. 2014;17(6):515–50; discussion 50.

10. Deer TR, Mekhail N, Provenzano D, Pope J, Krames E, Thomson S, et al. The appropriate use of neurostimulation: avoidance and treatment of complications of neurostimulation therapies for the treatment of chronic pain. Neuromodulation : J Int Neuromodulation Soc. 2014; 17(6):571–97; discussion 97–8.
11. Alo KM. Lead positioning and programming strategies in the treatment of complex pain. Neuromodulation : J Int Neuromodulation Soc. 1999;2(3):165–70.
12. Kumar K, Caraway DL, Rizvi S, Bishop S. Current challenges in spinal cord stimulation. Neuromodulation: J Int Neuromodulation Soc. 2014;17 Suppl 1:22–35.
13. Levy RM. Anatomic considerations for spinal cord stimulation. Neuromodulation: J Int Neuromodulation Soc. 2014;17 Suppl 1:2–11.
14. Holsheimer J, den Boer JA, Struijk JJ, Rozeboom AR. MR assessment of the normal position of the spinal cord in the spinal canal. AJNR Am J Neuroradiol. 1994;15(5):951–9.